My Daily Alkaline Smoothie

A Complete Illustrated Guide for Your Healthy Alkaline Smoothies

Naomi Whiteley

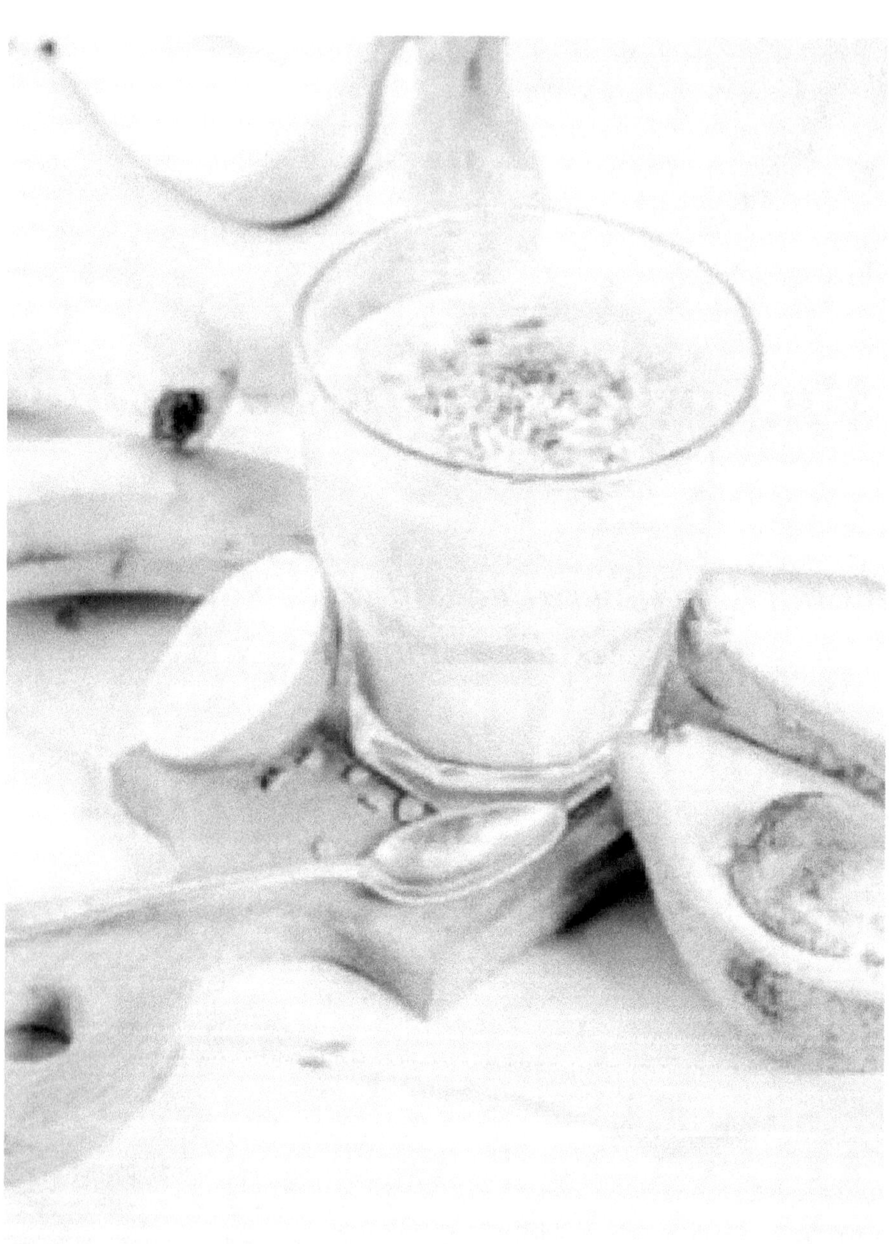

professional before attempting any techniques outlined in this book.

By reading this document, the reader agrees that under no circumstances is the author responsible for any losses, direct or indirect, which are incurred as a result of the use of information contained within this document, including, but not limited to, — errors, omissions, or inaccuracies.

Table of Contents

FROZEN SUN SMOOTHIE...7

BELL PEPPER SMOOTHIE...9

NUTTY APPLE SMOOTHIE...11

BLUEBERRY BREAKFAST SMOOTHIE...13

SWEET GREEN SMOOTHIE...15

GREEN-MIX SMOOTHIE...17

PERFECT LUNCH SMOOTHIE..19

PEACH SMOOTHIE..21

BLUEBERRY AROMA SMOOTHIE...23

LIVER DETOX SMOOTHIE...25

CHERRY SMOOTHIE...27

FRESH ZUCCHINI SMOOTHIE...29

BANANA-PEAR SMOOTHIE..31

SMOOTHIE WITH ARUGULA..33

SUMMER SMOOTHIE...35

PURE CACTUS SMOOTHIE...37

BLACK CURRANT SMOOTHIE..39

RASPBERRY SMOOTHIE..41

PURE MANGO SMOOTHIE...43

TAMARIND SMOOTHIE...45

INGREDIENTS:...45

LIGHT SMOOTHIE...47

PEAR AND GRAPE SMOOTHIE...49

ICE BLUEBERRY SMOOTHIE..51

APPLE AND AVOCADO SMOOTHIE...53

KAMUT SMOOTHIE...55

GARBANZO BEANS SMOOTHIE...57

Sweet Cucumber Smoothie 59

Nori Smoothie 61

Prickly Pear Smoothie 63

Pure Avocado Smoothie 65

Recovery Smoothie 67

Soursops Smoothie 69

Ocean Blue Smoothie 71

Tomato Smoothie 73

Berryland Smoothie 75

Green Tonic Smoothie 77

Hearty Smoothie 79

Dulse Smoothie 81

Anti-Cholesterol Smoothie 83

Anti-Inflammation Smoothie 85

Heart-Healthy Smoothie 87

Purslane Smoothie 89

Anti-Allergy Smoothie 91

Three-Berry Smoothie 93

Ice Cream Smoothie 95

Lettuce Smoothie 97

Aid Digestion Smoothie 99

One-Third Smoothie 101

Squash Smoothie 103

Nutty Date Smoothie 105

Frozen Sun Smoothie

Ingredients:

Melons (Seeded), 9 oz (255 g)

Date Sugar, 2 teaspoons

Ice, cubed, ½ cup

Instructions:

1. Cut melon for the blender.

2. Blend all ingredients in a high-speed blender until smooth.

3. Enjoy!

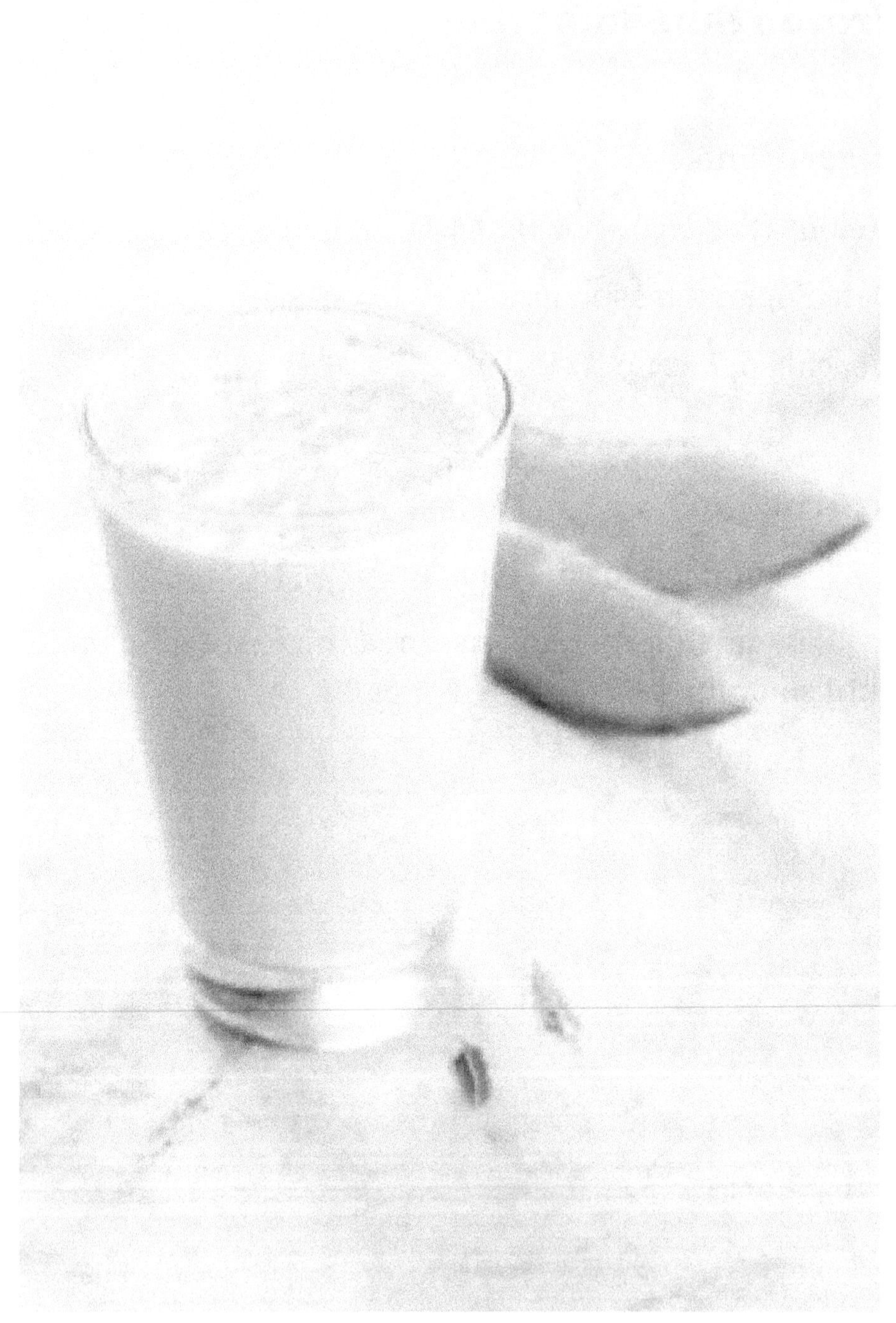

Bell Pepper Smoothie

Ingredients:

3 Bell Peppers

Date Sugar, 2 teaspoons

1 Bananas (The smallest one or the Burro/midsize/original banana)

Instructions:

1.   Cut banana and bell peppers for the blender.

2.   Blend all ingredients in a high-speed blender until smooth.

3.   Enjoy!

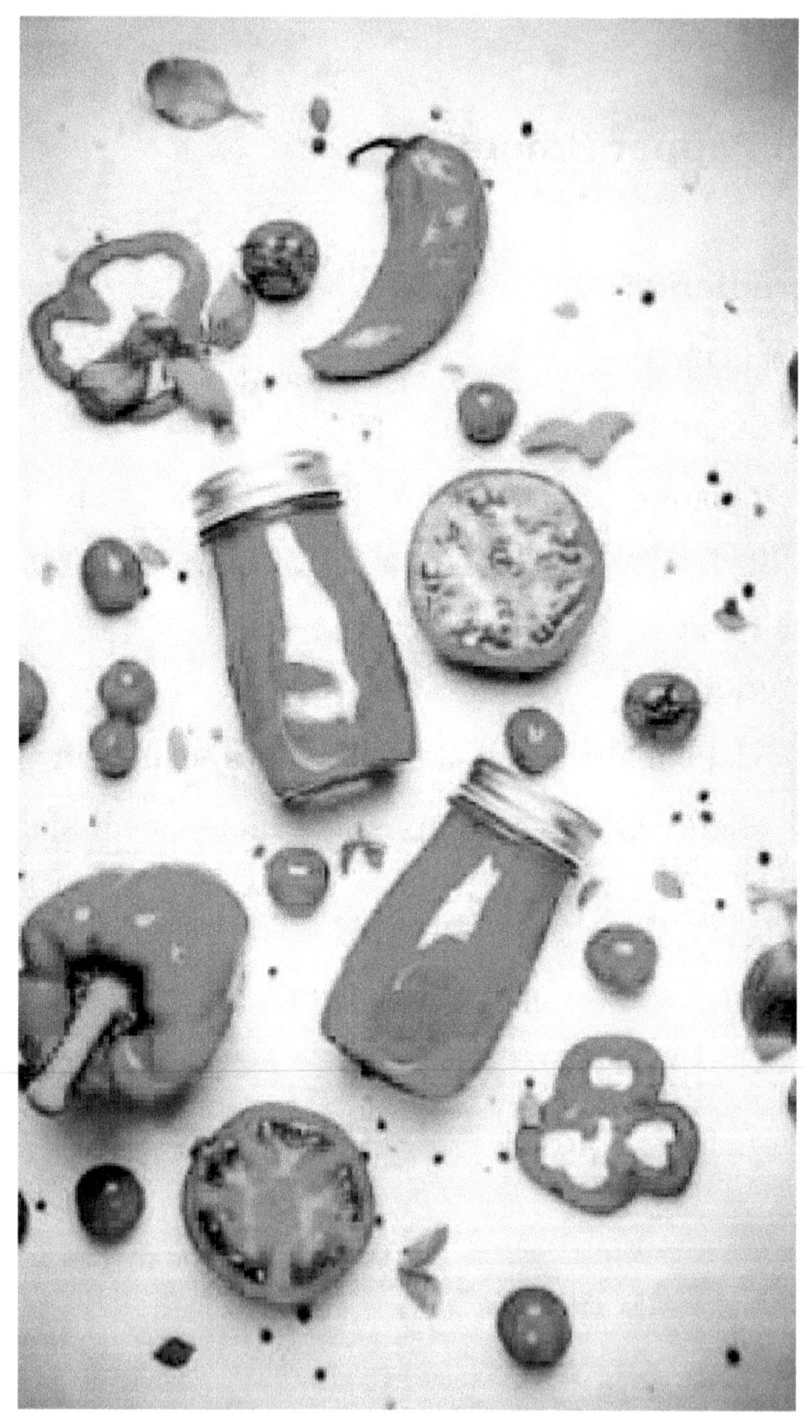

Nutty Apple Smoothie

Ingredients:

2 Apples, pitted

Date Sugar, 2 teaspoons

Brazil Nuts or Walnuts, ½ cup

Instructions:

1. Cut apples for the blender.

2. Blend all ingredients in a high-speed blender until smooth.

3. Enjoy!

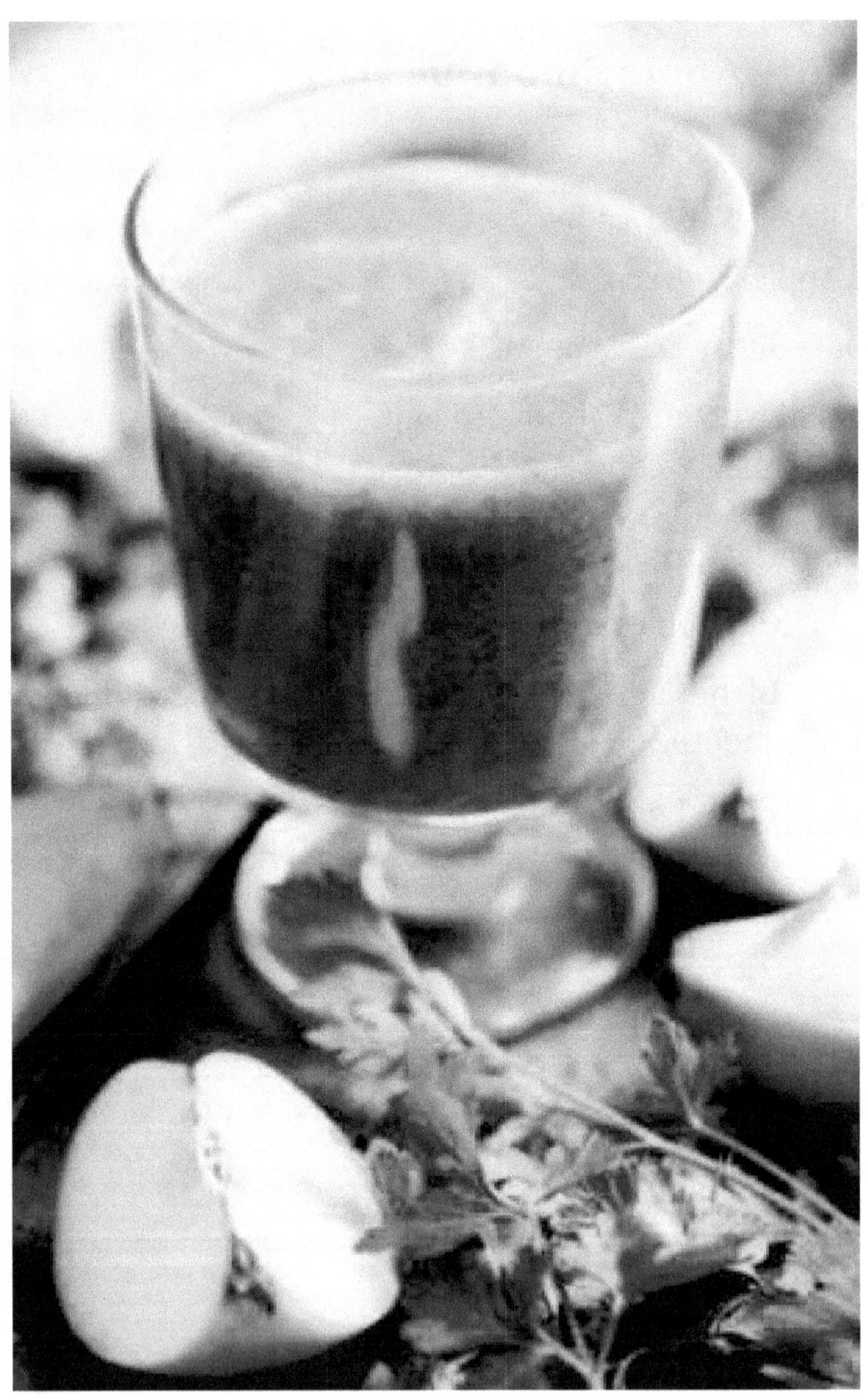

Blueberry Breakfast Smoothie

Ingredients:

Soft Jelly Coconut Milk (or homemade walnut milk), ¼ cup

Date Sugar, 2 teaspoons

Blueberries, ½ cup

Brazil Nuts or Walnuts, ½ cup

Instructions:

1.   Blend all ingredients in a high-speed blender until smooth.

2.   Enjoy!

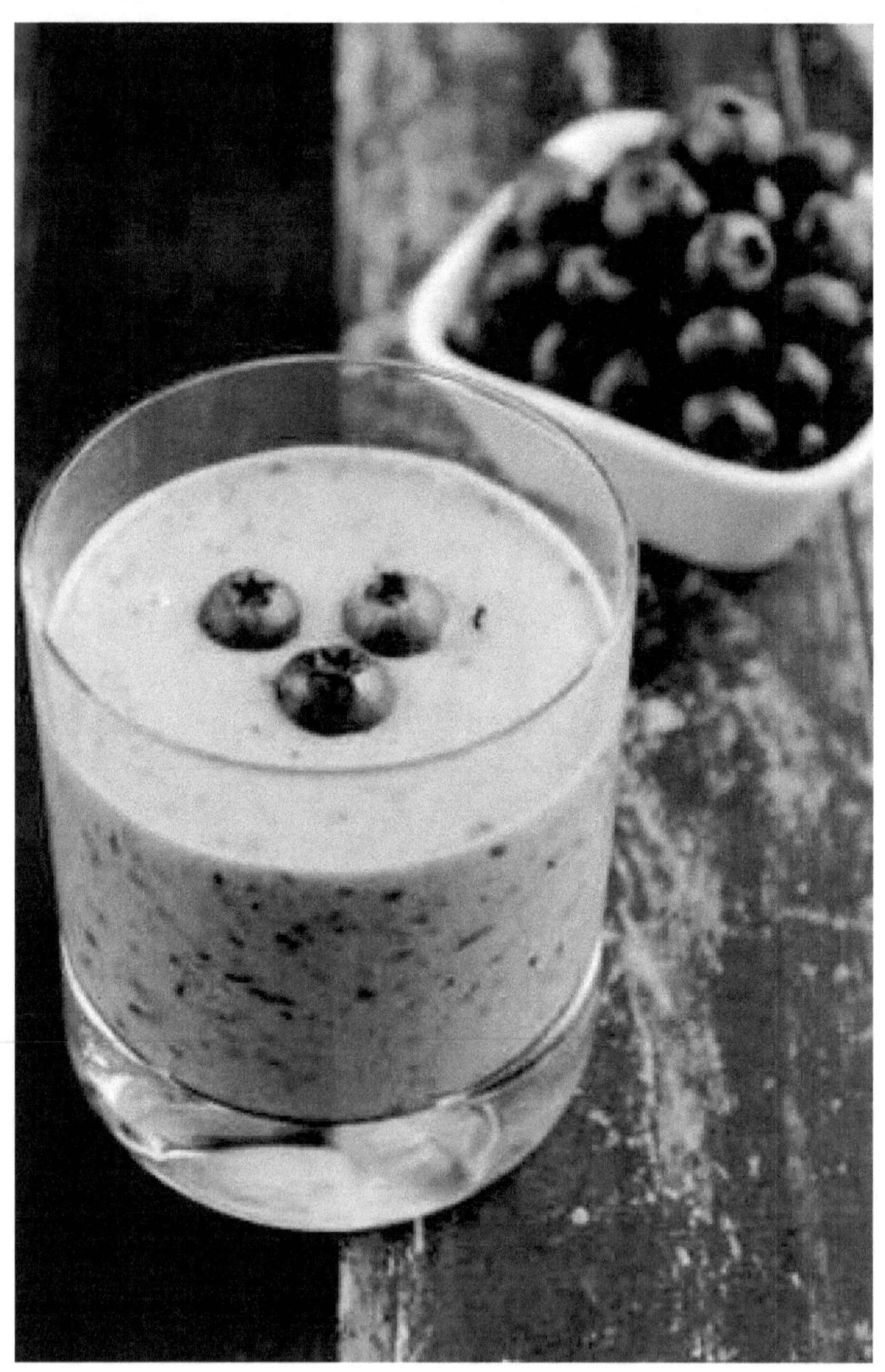

Sweet Green Smoothie

Ingredients:

2 Cucumber

2 Apples, pitted

Date Sugar, 3 teaspoons

Basil, About 4 leaves

Instructions:

1.   Cut apples and cucumbers for the blender.

2.   Blend all ingredients in a high-speed blender until smooth.

3.   Enjoy!

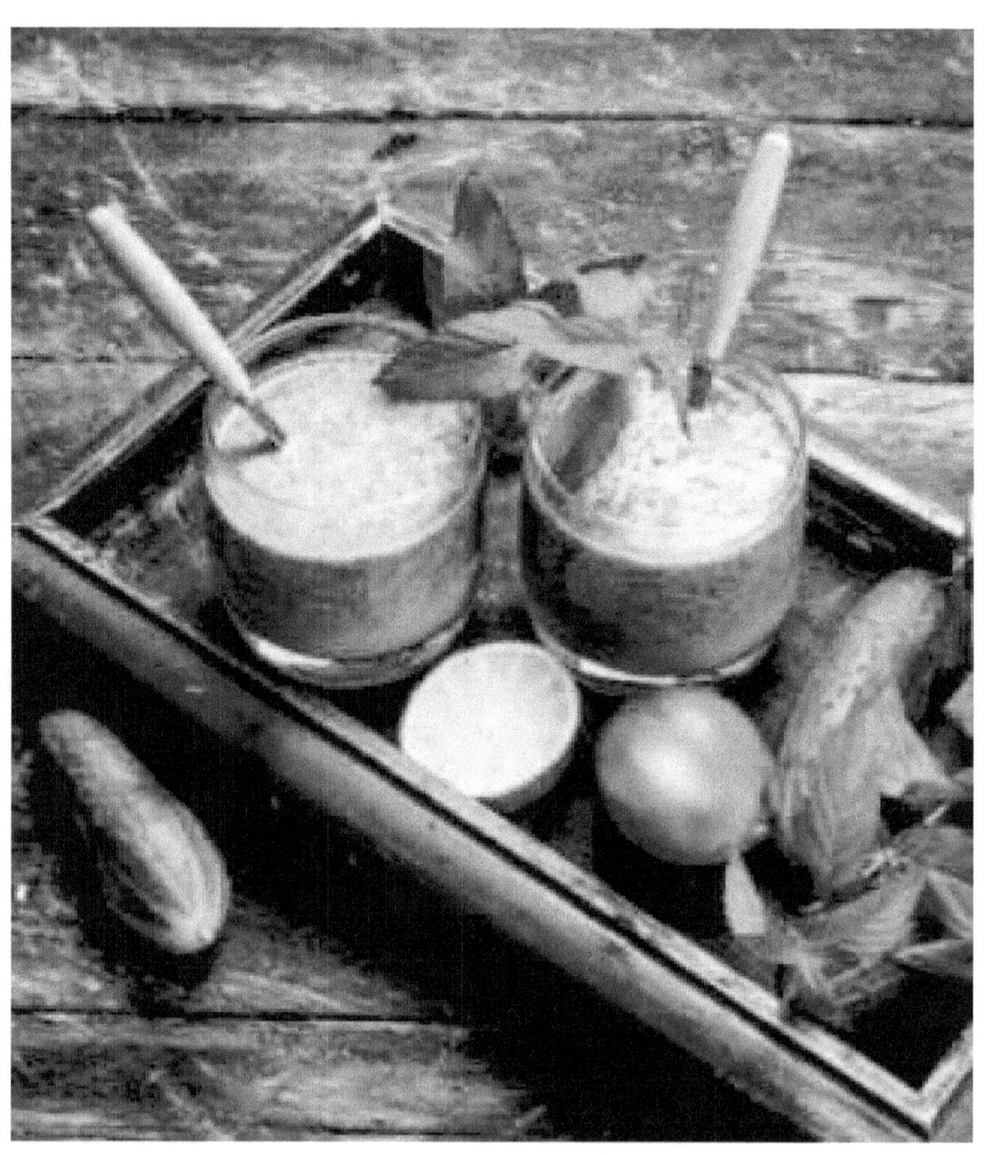

Green-Mix Smoothie

Ingredients:

½ Avocado, peeled, pitted

Lime juice, 1 teaspoon

Kale leaves, chopped, ½ cup

Raw Sesame Seeds, 2 tablespoon

Instructions:

1.   Cut avocado for the blender.

2.   Blend all ingredients in a high-speed blender until smooth.

3.   Enjoy!

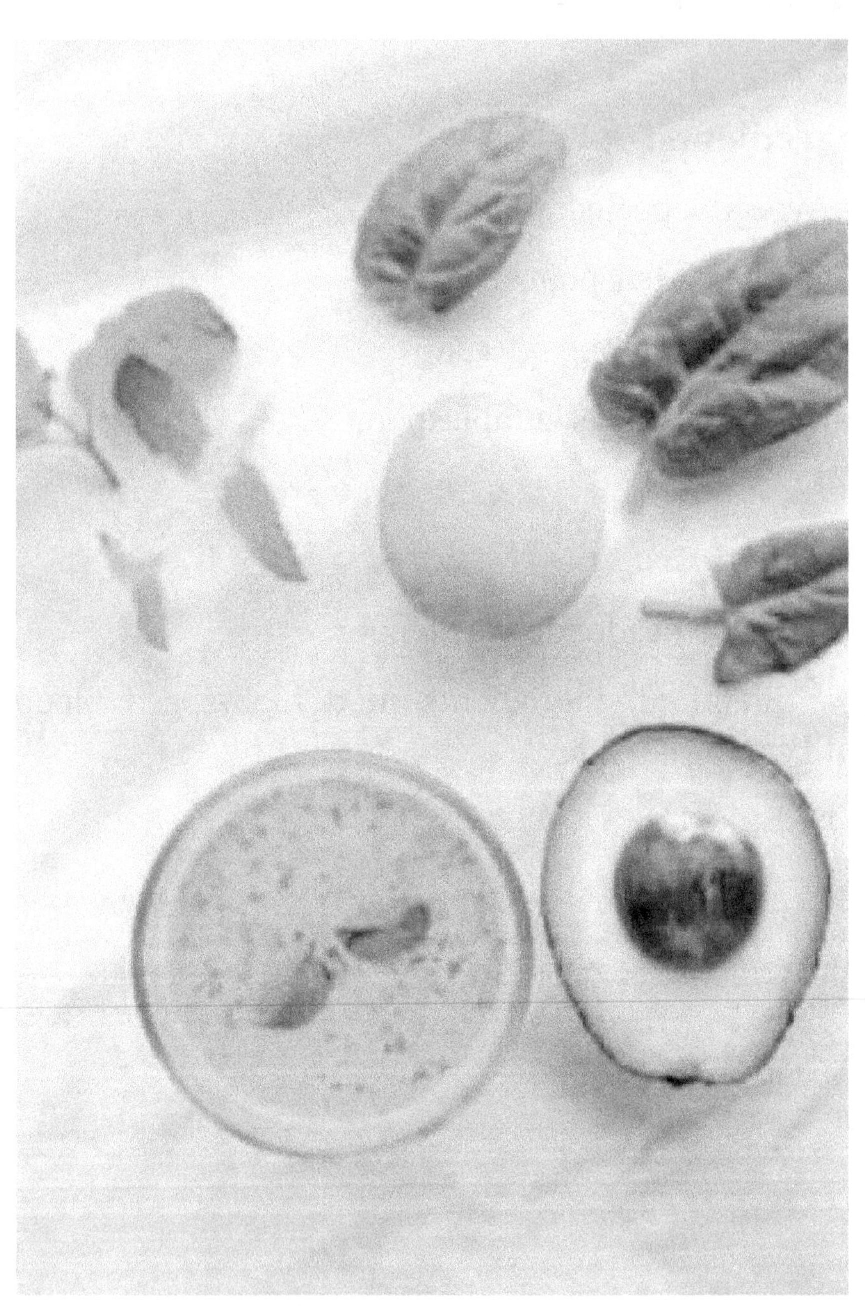

Perfect Lunch Smoothie

Ingredients:

½ Avocado, peeled, pitted

Date Sugar, 2 teaspoons

Raw Sesame Seeds, 1 tablespoon

2 Bananas (The smallest one or the Burro/midsize/original banana)

Instructions:

1. Cut bananas and avocado for the blender.

2. Blend all ingredients in a high-speed blender until smooth.

3. Enjoy!

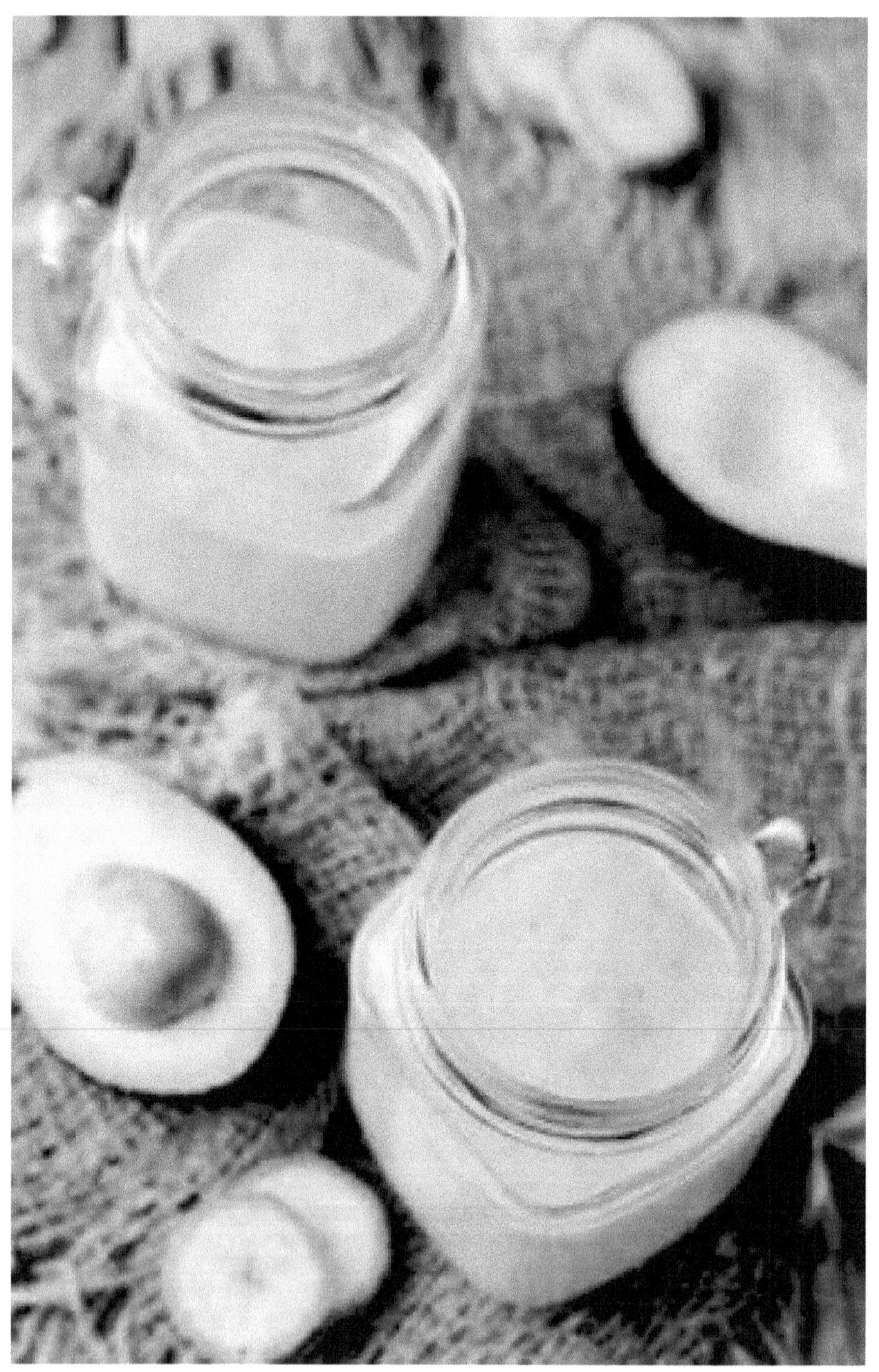

Peach Smoothie

Ingredients:

4 Peaches, pitted

2 Bananas (The smallest one or the Burro/midsize/original banana)

Instructions:

1.   Cut bananas and peaches for the blender.

2.   Blend all ingredients in a high-speed blender until smooth.

3.   Enjoy!

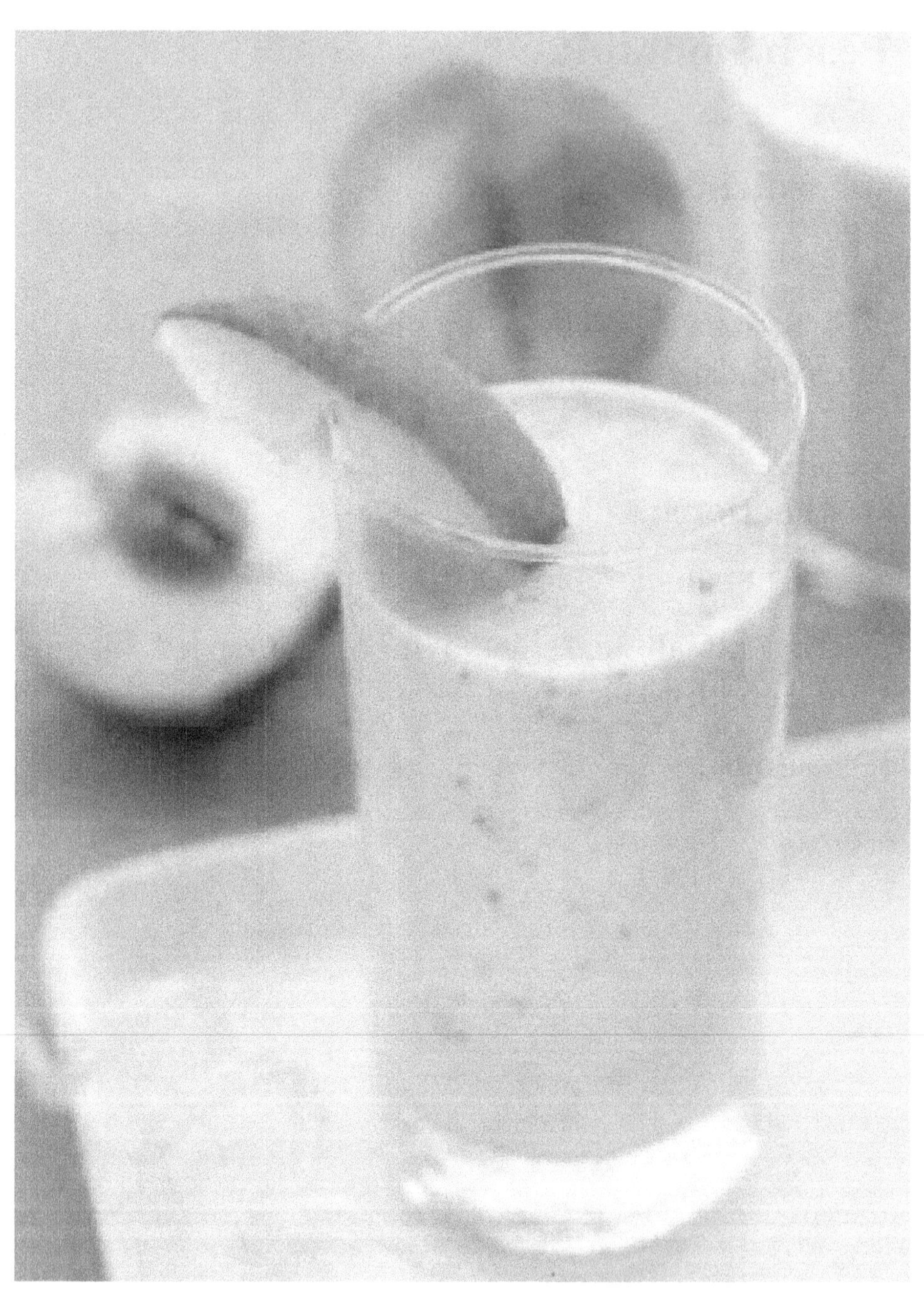

Blueberry Aroma Smoothie

Ingredients:

Date Sugar, 2 teaspoons

Ice, cubed, ½ cup

Grapes (Seeded), ½ cup

Blueberries, ¼ cup

Instructions:

1.   Blend all ingredients in a high-speed blender until smooth.

2.   Enjoy!

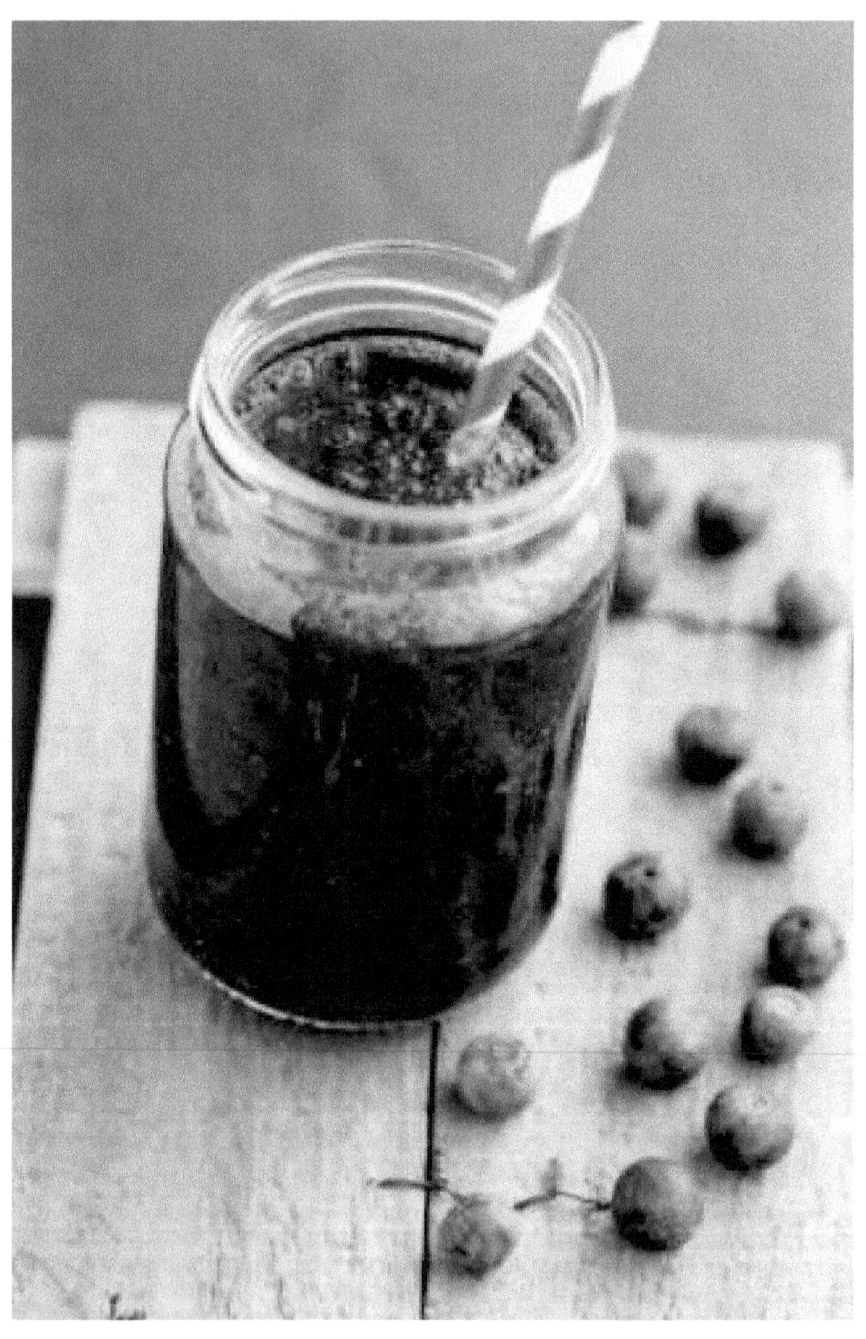

Liver Detox Smoothie

Ingredients:

Chamomile tea, ¼ cup

 ½ Avocado, peeled, pitted

Date Sugar, 2 teaspoons

Dandelion greens, ½ cup

2 Bananas (The smallest one or the Burro/midsize/original banana)

Instructions:

1. Boil ¼ cup of water. Add ½ teaspoon of chamomile and let it steep for 10-15 minutes.

2. Strain and let it cool.

3. Cut bananas and avocado for the blender.

4. Blend all ingredients in a high-speed blender until smooth.

5. Enjoy!

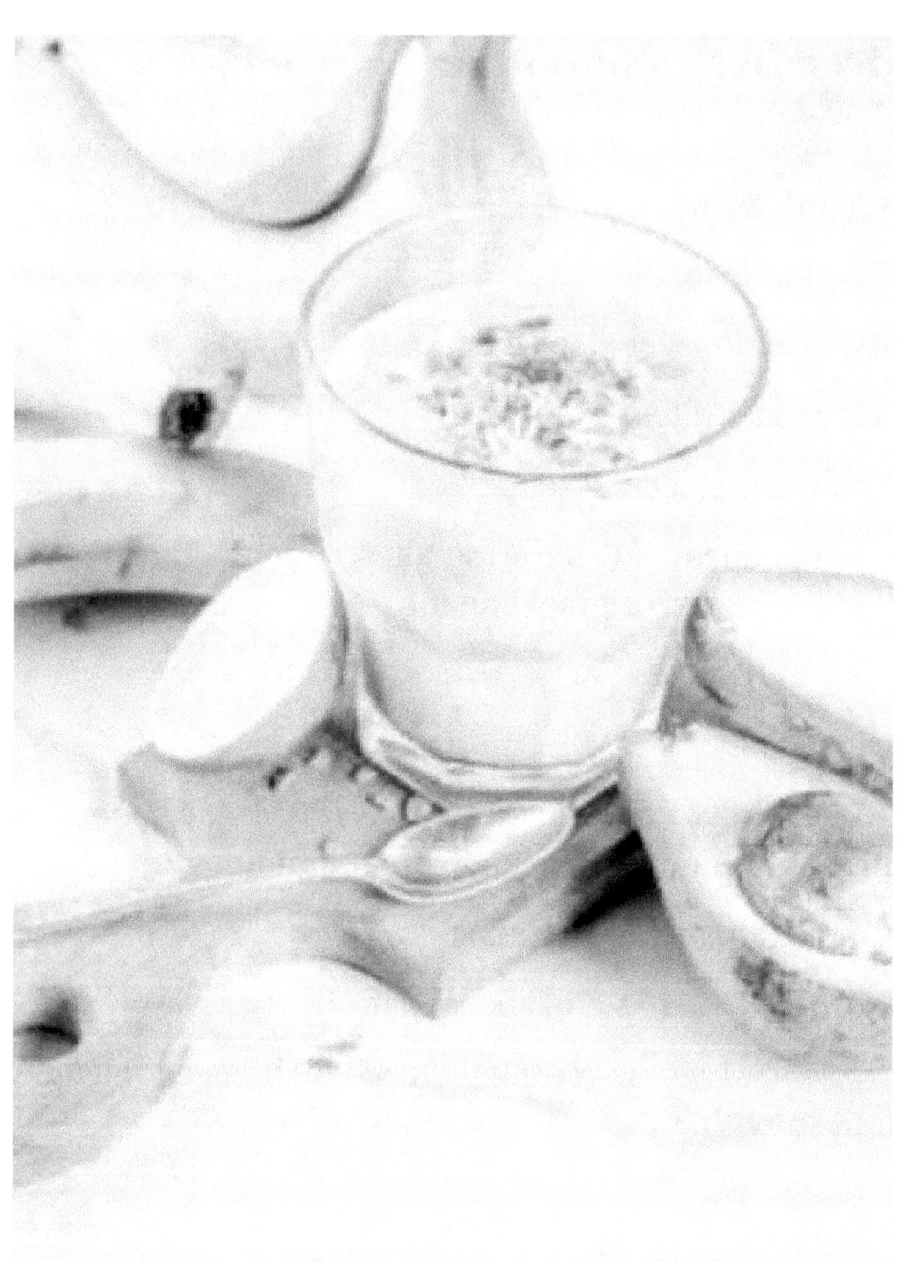

Cherry Smoothie

Ingredients:

Soft Jelly Coconut Milk (or homemade walnut milk), ½ cup

Date Sugar, 3 teaspoons

Cherries, pitted, ½ cup

Instructions:

1.   Blend all ingredients in a high-speed blender until smooth.

2.   Enjoy!

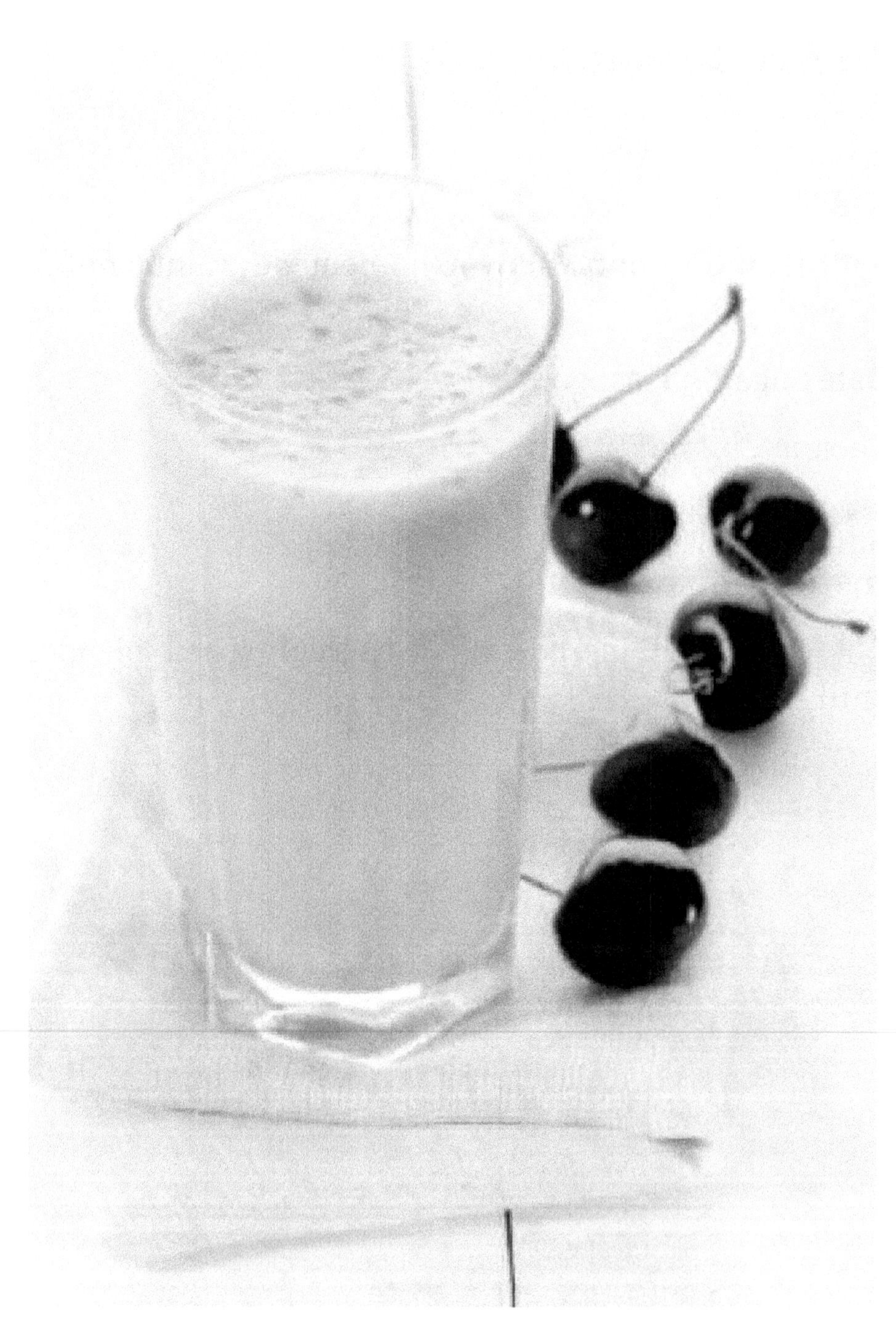

Fresh Zucchini Smoothie

Ingredients:

1 Zucchini

½ Avocado, peeled, pitted

Date Sugar, 2 teaspoons

Lime juice, 1 teaspoon

Fonio or Quinoa, cooked, ½ cup

Instructions:

1.	Cut zucchini and avocado for the blender.

2.	Blend all ingredients in a high-speed blender until smooth.

3.	Enjoy!

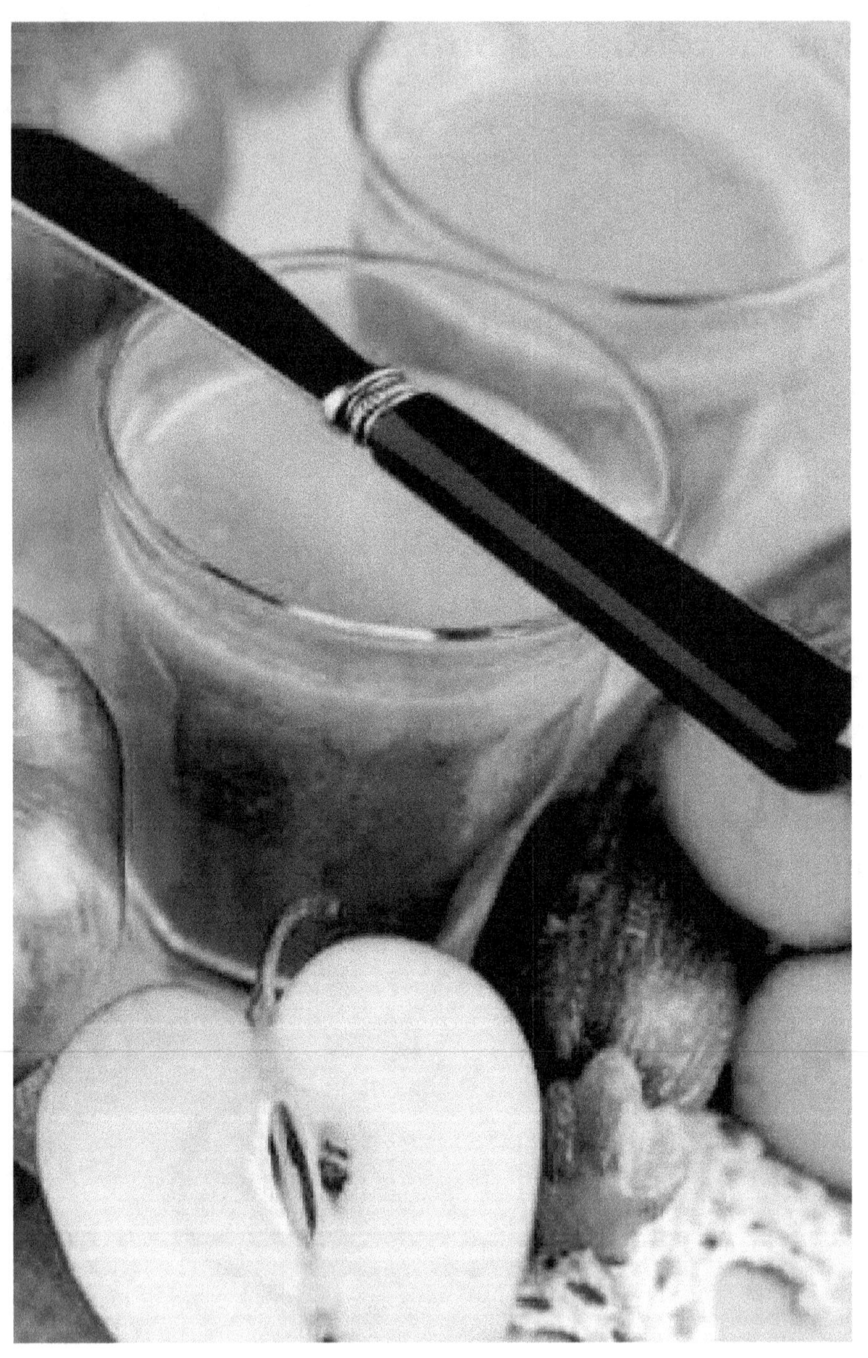

Banana-Pear Smoothie

Ingredients:

2 Pears, pitted

3 Bananas (The smallest one or the Burro/midsize/original banana)

Instructions:

1. Cut bananas and pears for the blender.

2. Blend all ingredients in a high-speed blender until smooth.

3. Enjoy!

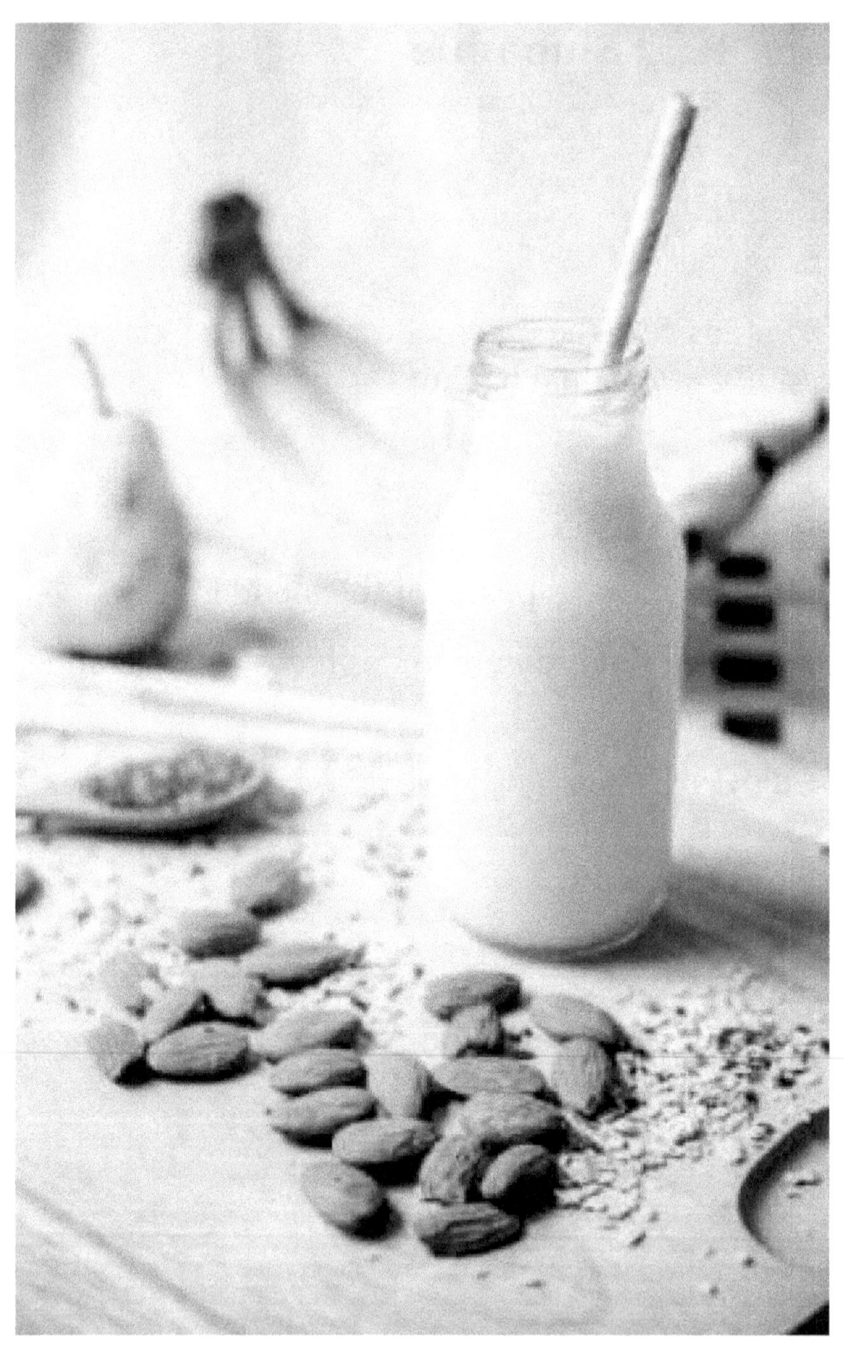

Smoothie with Arugula

Ingredients:

Soft Jelly Coconut Milk (or homemade walnut milk), ¼ cup

Date Sugar, 2 teaspoons

Wild Arugula, ½ cup

2 Apples, pitted

Instructions:

1.   Cut apples for the blender.

2.   Blend all ingredients in a high-speed blender until smooth.

3.   Enjoy!

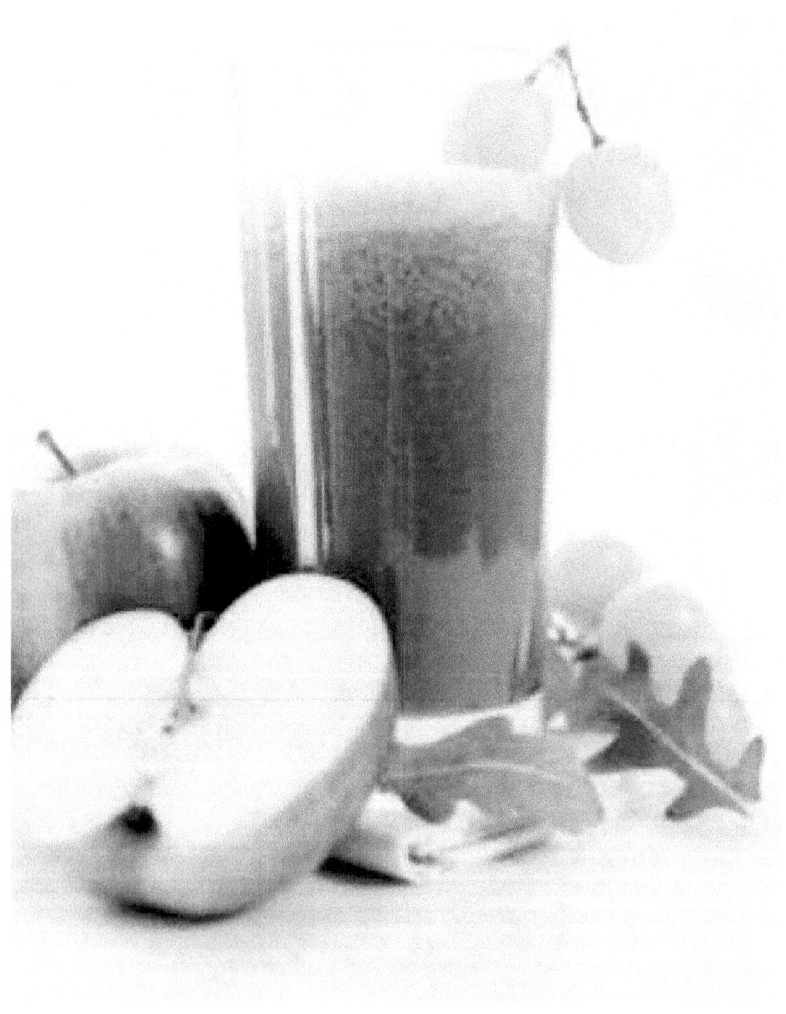

Summer Smoothie

Ingredients:

Cantaloupe, 7 oz (198 g)

2 Bananas (The smallest one or the Burro/midsize/original banana)

Instructions:

1. Cut bananas and cantaloupe for the blender.

2. Blend all ingredients in a high-speed blender until smooth.

3. Enjoy!

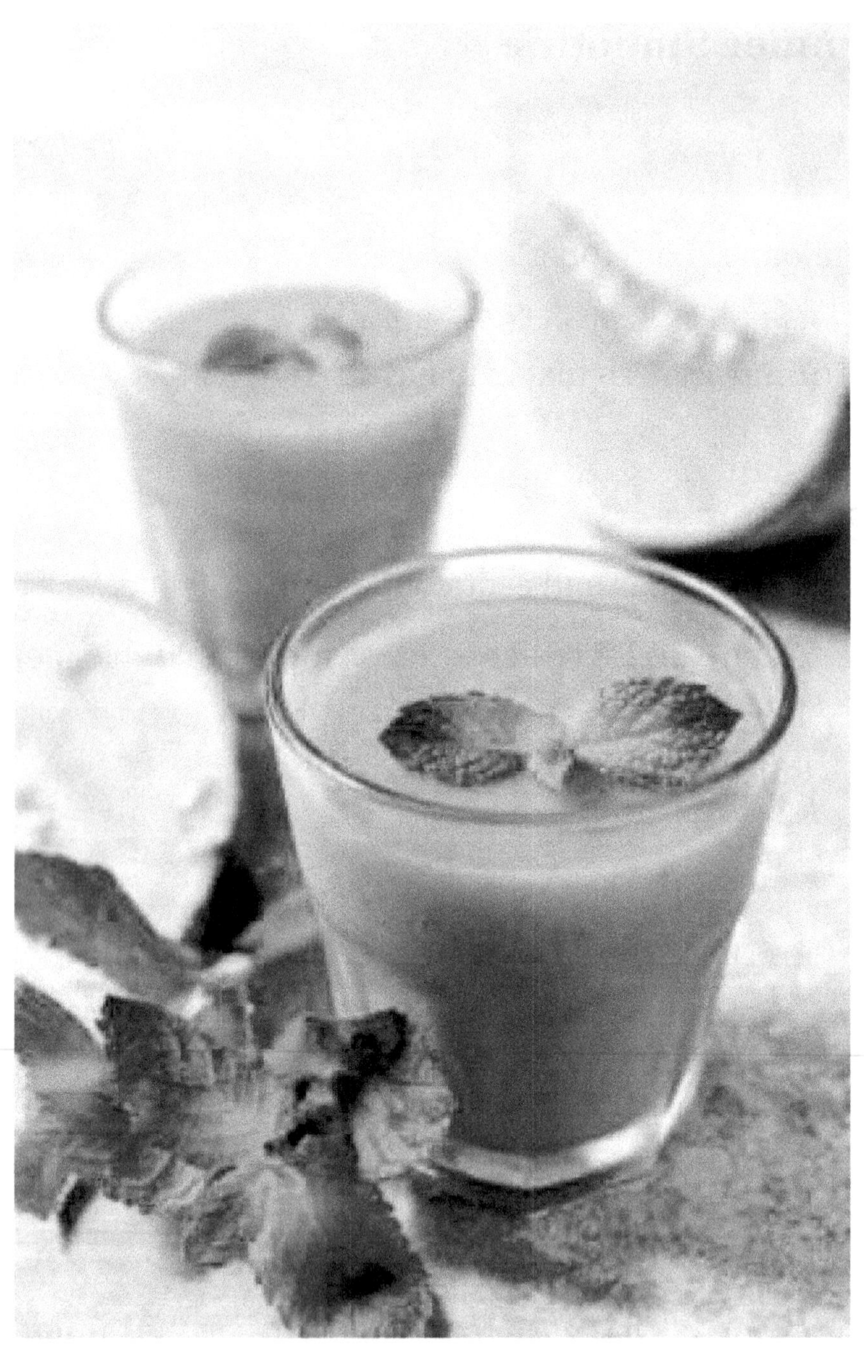

Pure Cactus Smoothie

Ingredients:

Izote (Cactus leaf), 1 cup

Lime juice, 1 teaspoon

Instructions:

1.	Cut cactus leaves for the blender.

2.	Blend all ingredients in a high-speed blender until smooth.

3.	Enjoy!

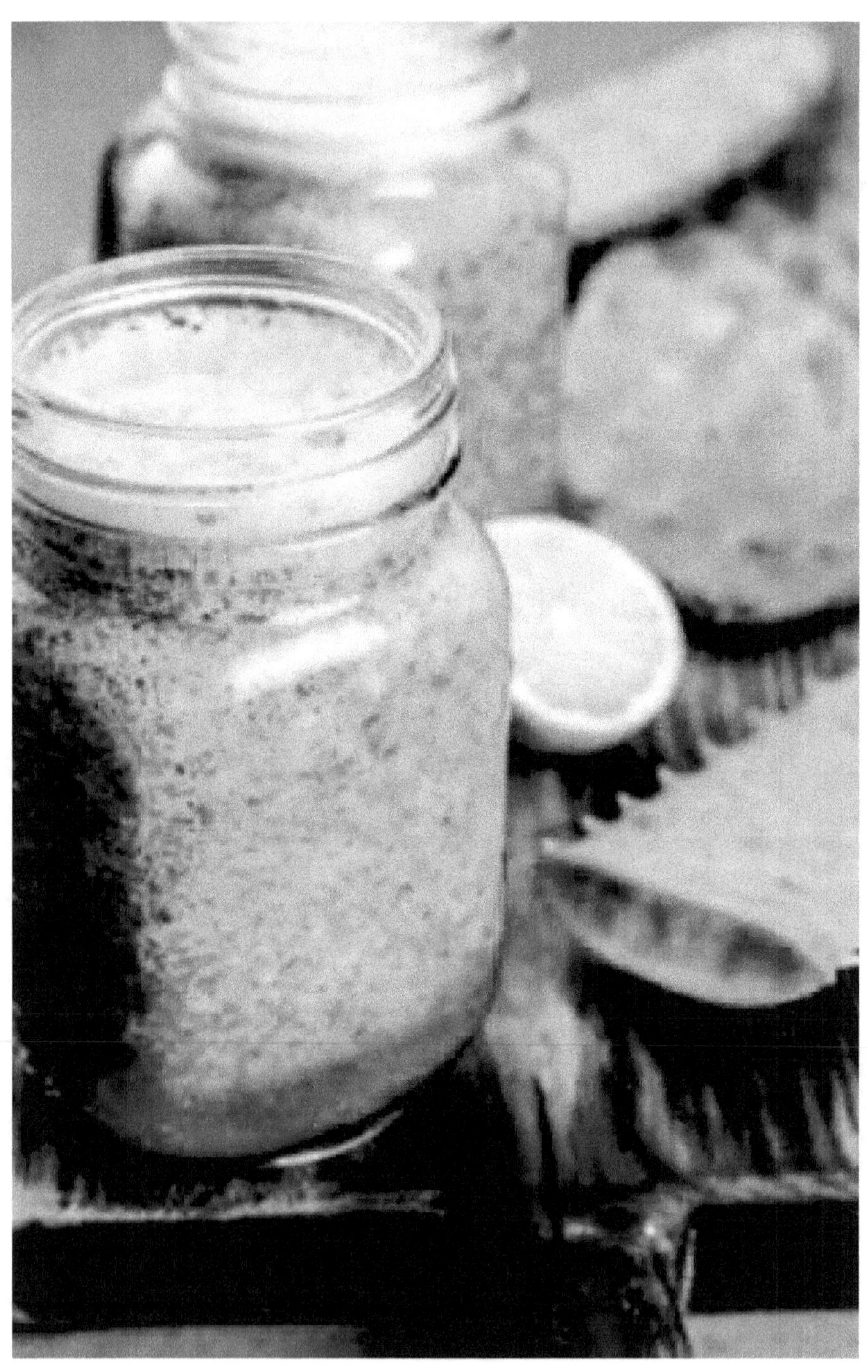

Black Currant Smoothie

Ingredients:

Soft Jelly Coconut Milk (or homemade walnut milk), ¼ cup

Date Sugar, 2 teaspoons

1, Bananas (The smallest one or the Burro/midsize/original banana)

Black Currants, ½ cup

Instructions:

1.   Cut banana for the blender.

2.   Blend all ingredients in a high-speed blender until smooth.

3.   Enjoy!

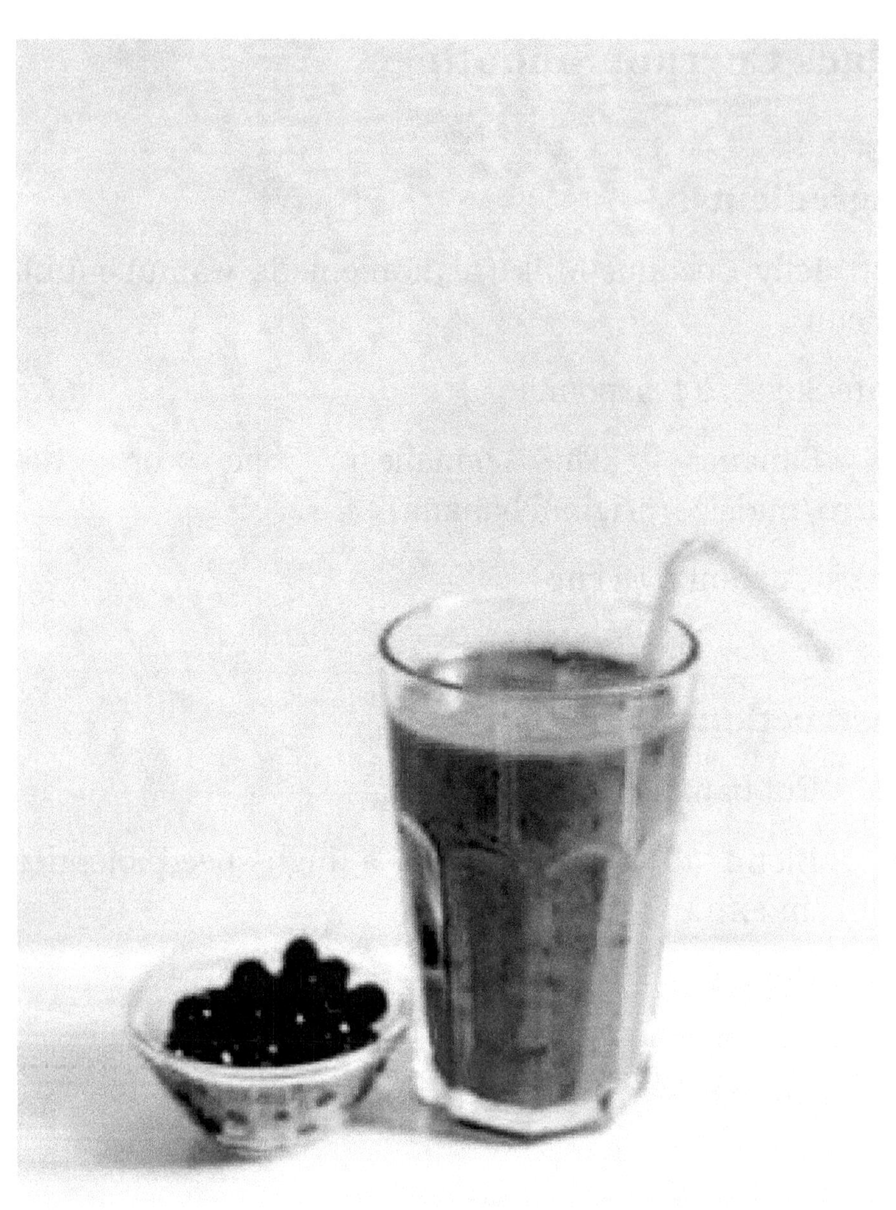

Raspberry Smoothie

Ingredients:

Soft Jelly Coconut Milk (or homemade walnut milk), ½ cup

Date Sugar, 2 teaspoons

Raspberries, ½ cup

1 Bananas (The smallest one or the Burro/midsize/original banana)

Instructions:

1. Cut banana for the blender.

2. Blend all ingredients in a high-speed blender until smooth.

3. Enjoy!

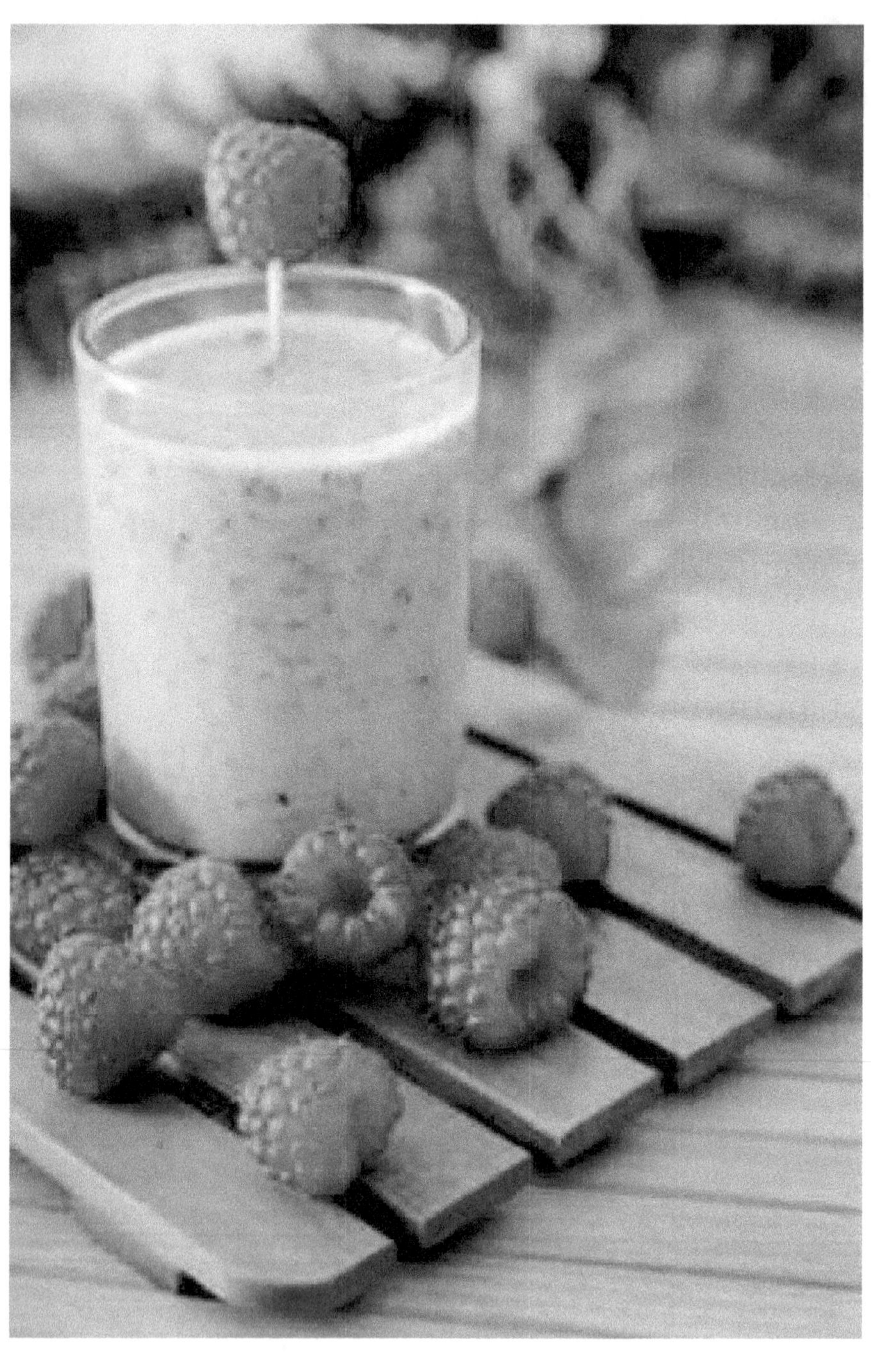

Pure Mango Smoothie

Ingredients:

1 Mango, peeled, pitted

1 Bananas (The smallest one or the Burro/midsize/original banana)

Chamomile tea, ¼ cup

Instructions:

1. Boil ¼ cup of water. Add ½ teaspoon of chamomile and let it steep for 10-15 minutes.

2. Cut banana and mango for the blender.

3. Blend all ingredients in a high-speed blender until smooth.

4. Enjoy!

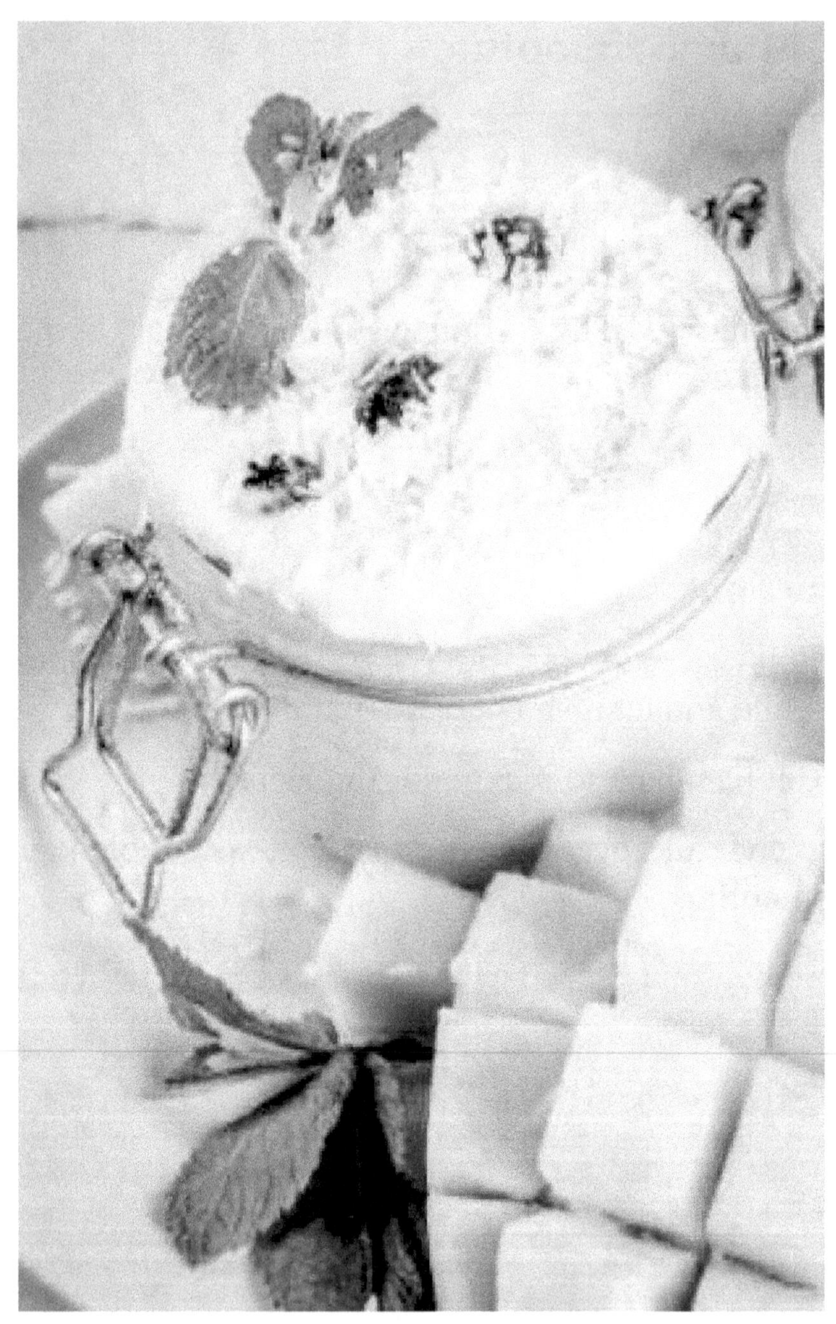

Tamarind Smoothie

Ingredients:

Soft Jelly Coconut Milk (or homemade walnut milk), ½ cup

Date Sugar, 2 teaspoons

1 Bananas (The smallest one or the Burro/midsize/original banana)

Tamarind, ½ cup

Instructions:

1.   Cut banana for the blender.

2.   Blend all ingredients in a high-speed blender until smooth.

3.   Enjoy!

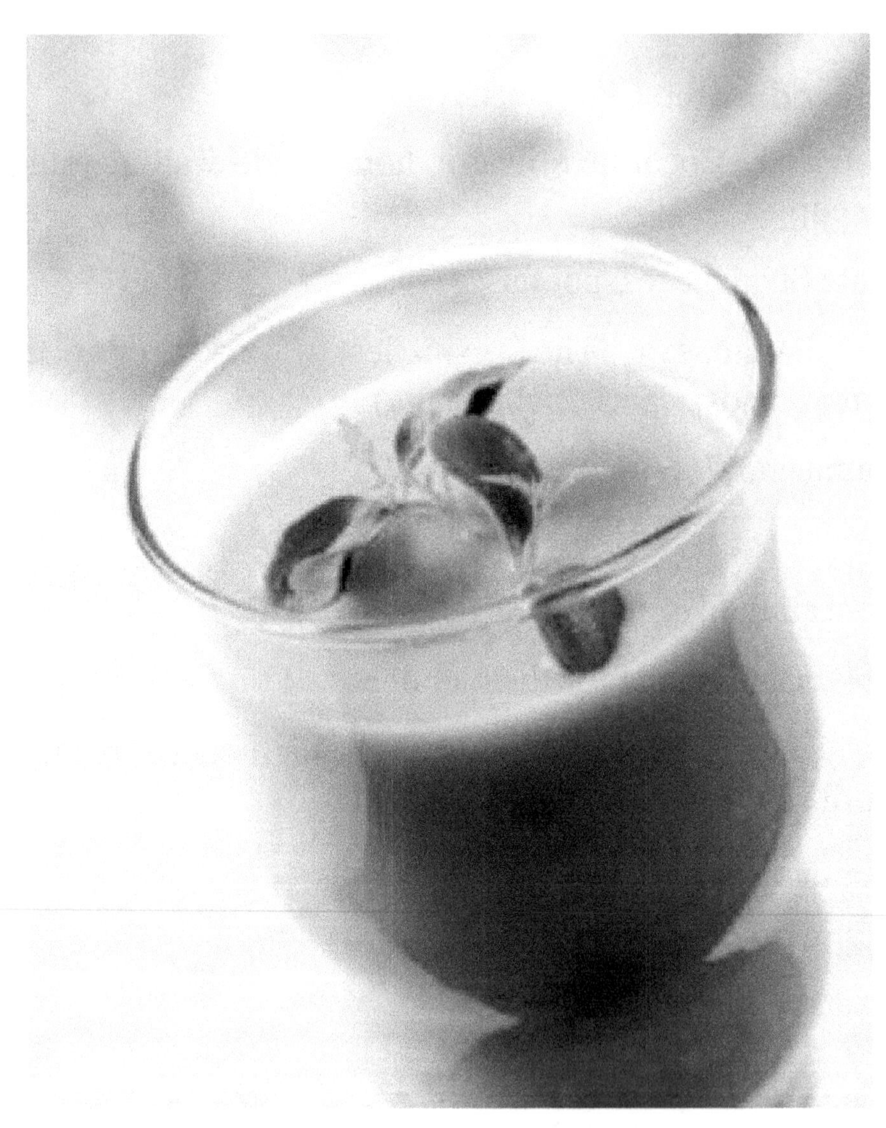

Light Smoothie

Ingredients:

Melons (Seeded), 10 oz (283 g)

Chamomile tea, ¼ cup

Date Sugar, 2 teaspoons

Instructions:

1. Boil ¼ cup of water. Add ½ teaspoon of chamomile and let it steep for 10-15 minutes.

2. Strain and let it cool.

3. Cut melon for the blender.

4. Blend all ingredients in a high-speed blender until smooth.

5. Enjoy!

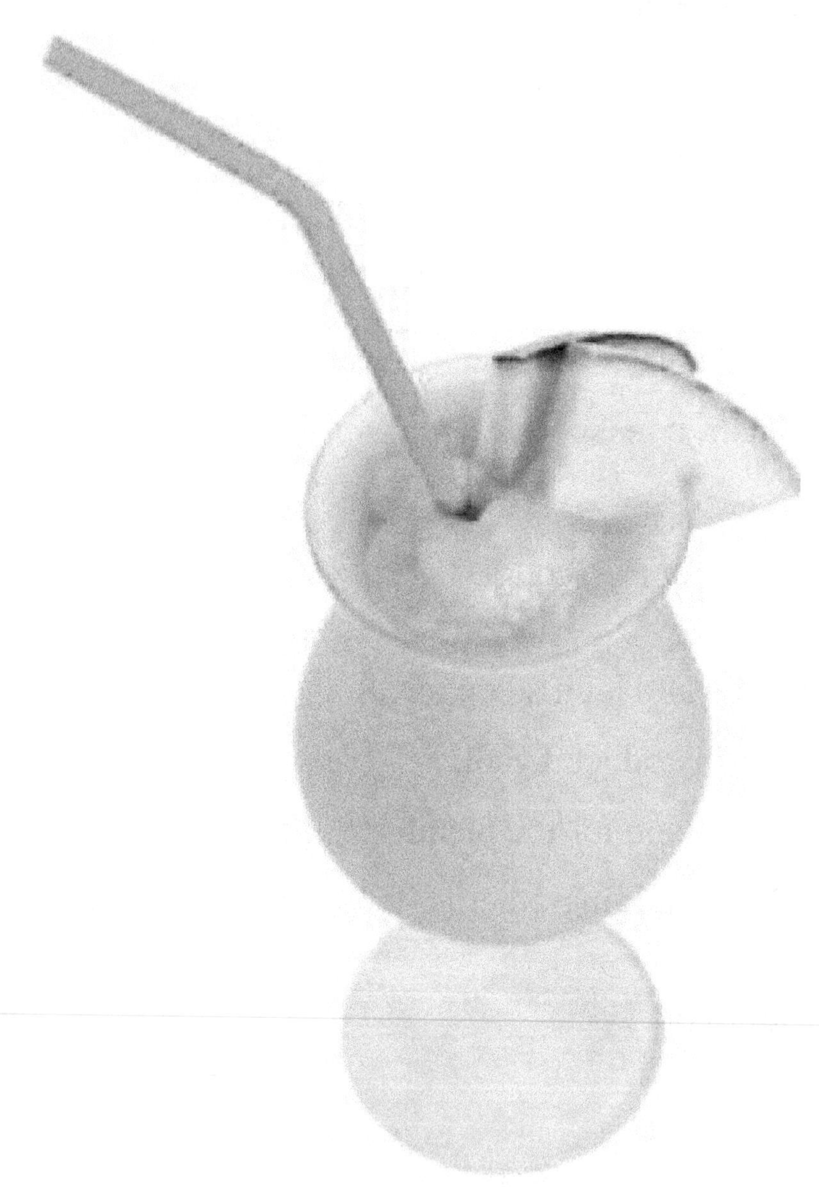

Pear and Grape Smoothie

Ingredients:

2 Pears, pitted

¼ cup Grapes (Seeded)

Instructions:

1.   Cut pears for the blender.

2.   Blend all ingredients in a high-speed blender until smooth.

3.   Enjoy!

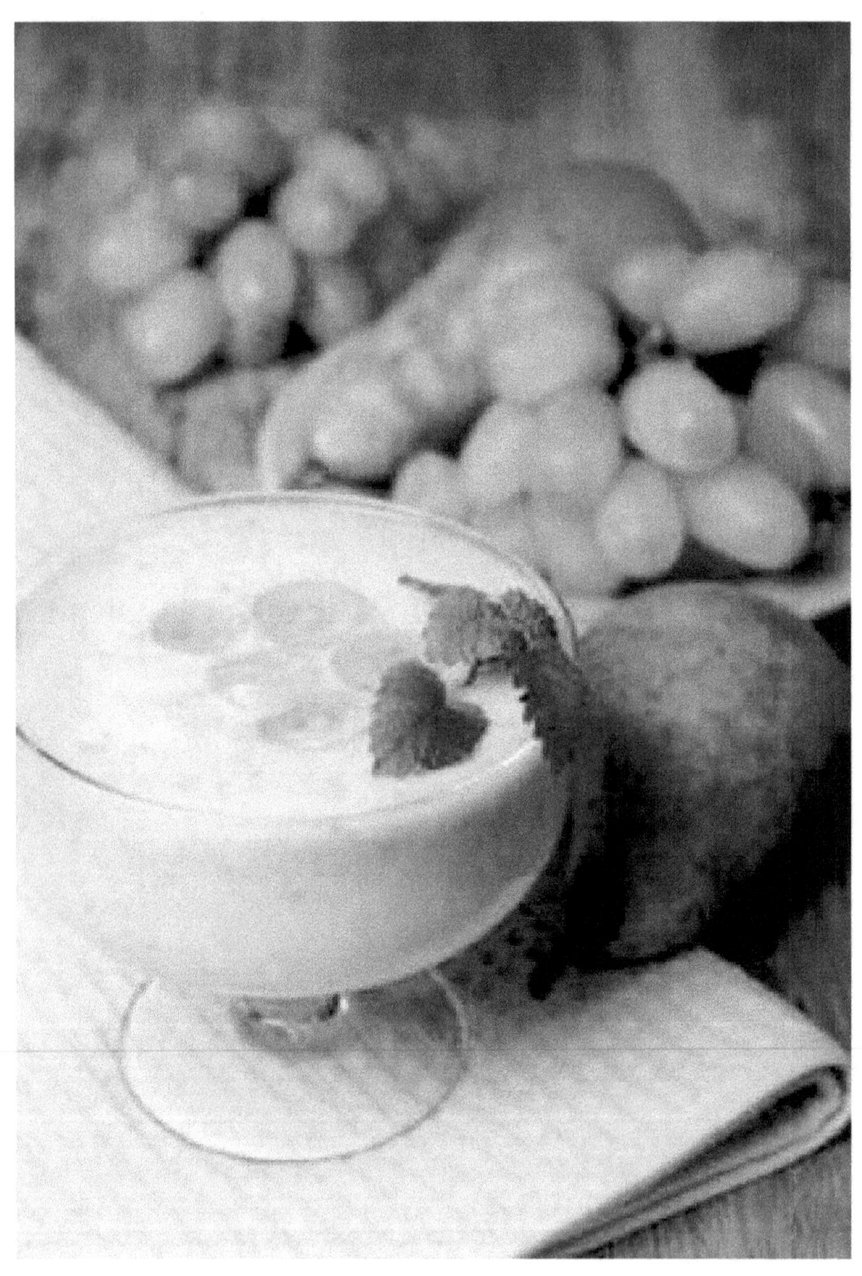

Ice Blueberry Smoothie

Ingredients:

Soft Jelly Coconut Milk (or homemade walnut milk), ¼ cup

Blueberries, ½ cup

Date Sugar, 2 teaspoons

Ice, cubed, ¼ cup

1 Bananas (The smallest one or the Burro/midsize/original banana)

Instructions:

1. Cut banana for the blender.

2. Blend all ingredients in a high-speed blender until smooth.

3. Enjoy!

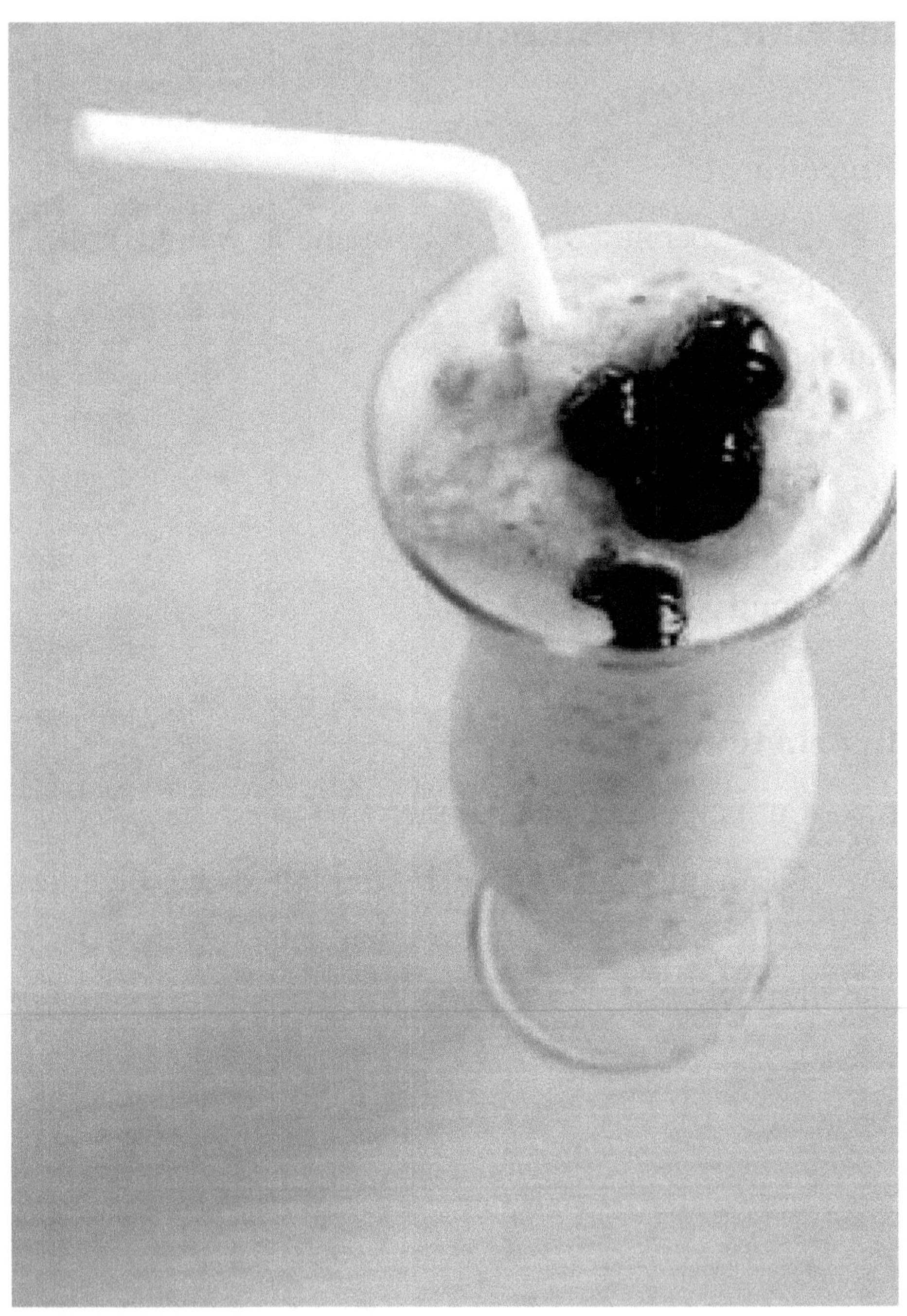

Apple and Avocado Smoothie

Ingredients:

Date Sugar, 2 teaspoons

½ Avocado, peeled, pitted

2 Apples, pitted

Instructions:

1.   Cut avocado and apples for the blender.

2.   Blend all ingredients in a high-speed blender until smooth.

3.   Enjoy!

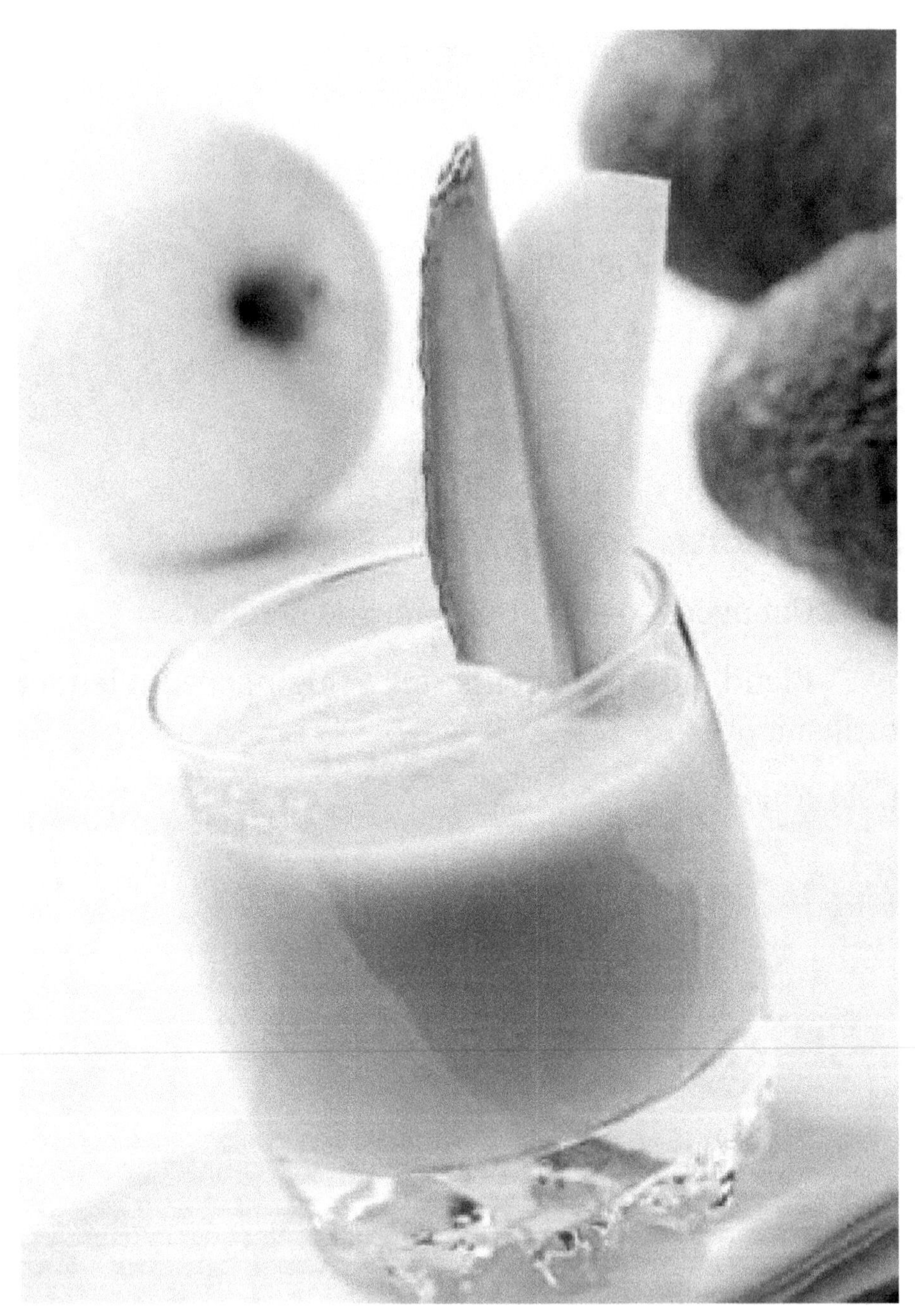

Kamut Smoothie

Ingredients:

Kamut, cooked, ¼ cup

Soft Jelly Coconut Milk (or homemade walnut milk), ½ cup

5 Dates, pitted

1 Bananas (The smallest one or the Burro/midsize/original banana)

Instructions:

1. Cut banana for the blender.

2. Blend all ingredients in a high-speed blender until smooth.

3. Enjoy!

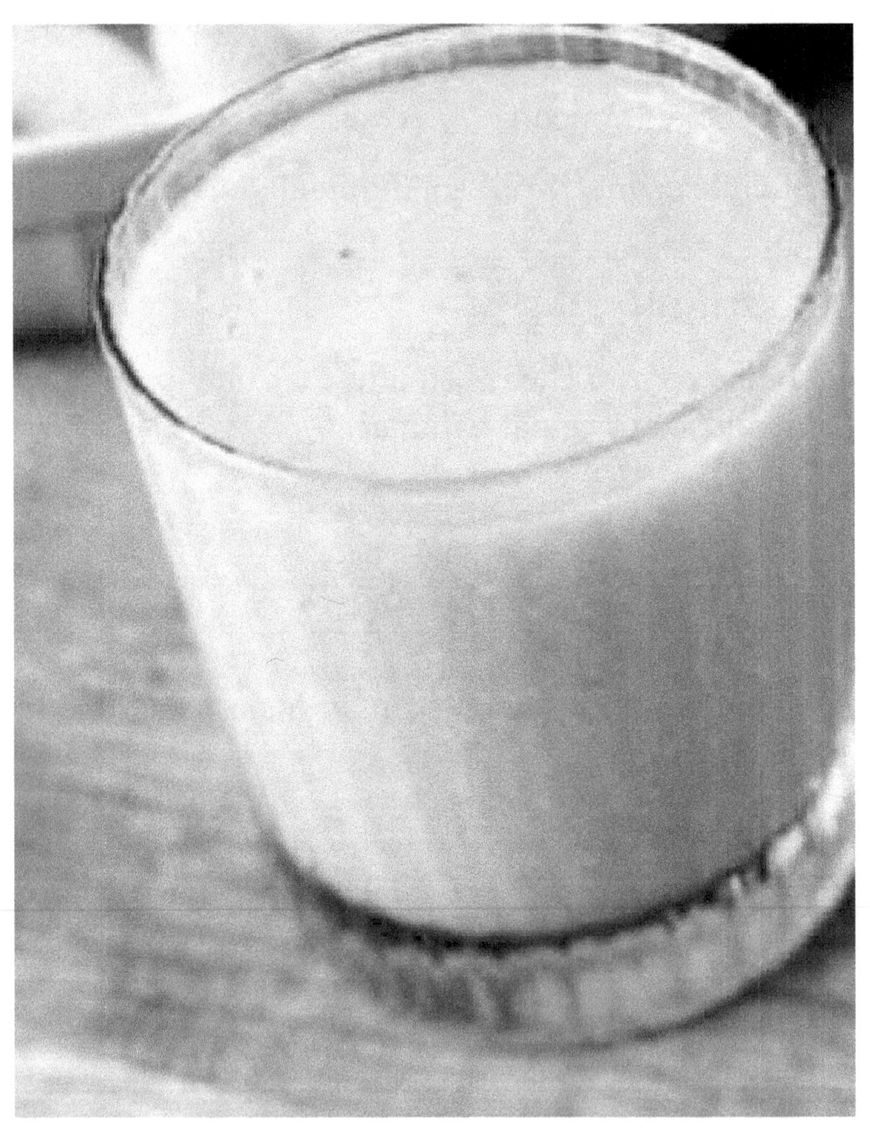

Garbanzo Beans Smoothie

Ingredients:

Garbanzo beans, cooked, ¼ cup

Soft Jelly Coconut Milk (or homemade walnut milk), ½ cup

5 Dates, pitted

1 Bananas (The smallest one or the Burro/midsize/original banana)

Instructions:

1. Cut banana for the blender.

2. Blend all ingredients in a high-speed blender until smooth.

3. Enjoy!

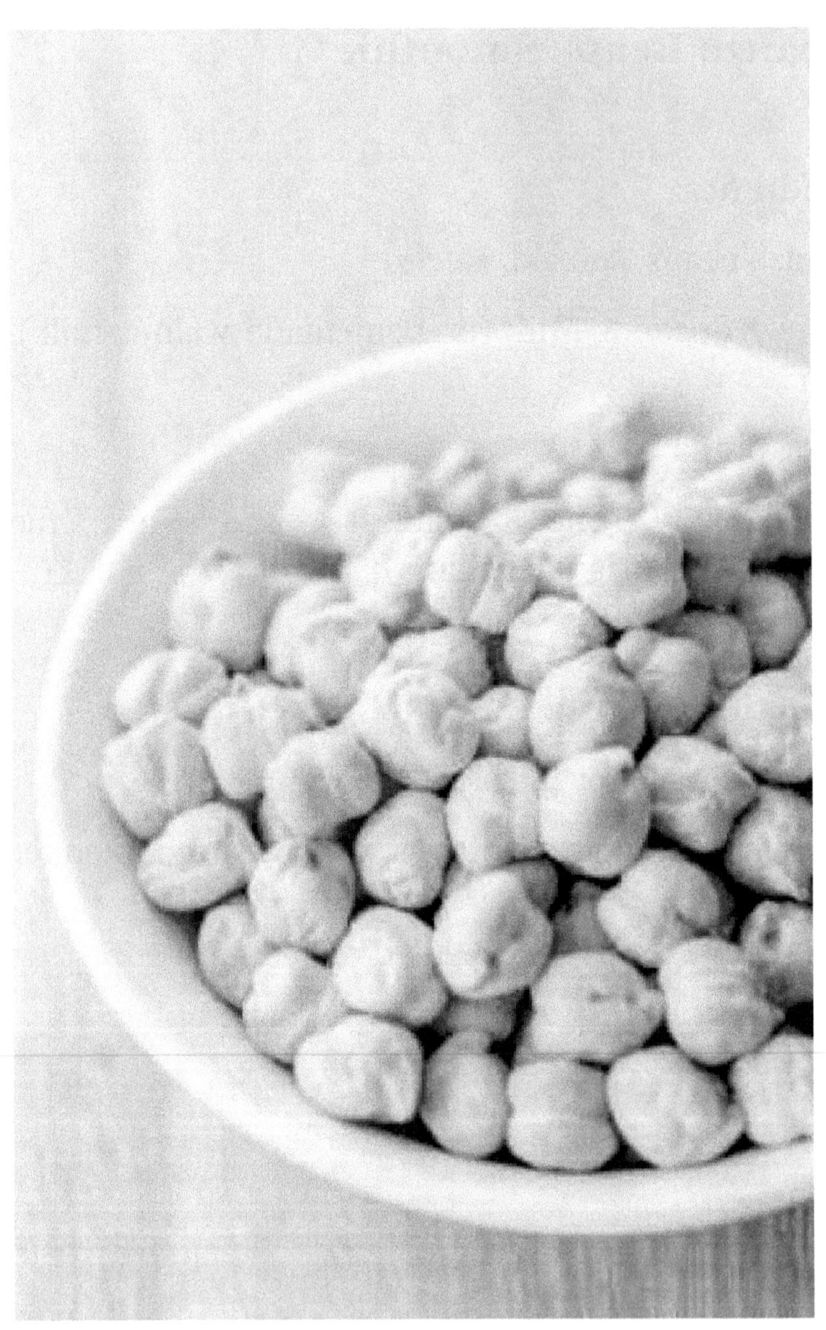

Sweet Cucumber Smoothie

Ingredients:

Basil 2 leaves

½ Avocado, peeled, pitted

2 Cucumber

Date Sugar, 2 teaspoons

Raw Sesame Seeds, 1 teaspoon

1 Bananas (The smallest one or the Burro/midsize/original banana)

Instructions:

1. Cut banana, avocado, and cucumbers for the blender.

2. Blend all ingredients in a high-speed blender until smooth.

3. Enjoy!

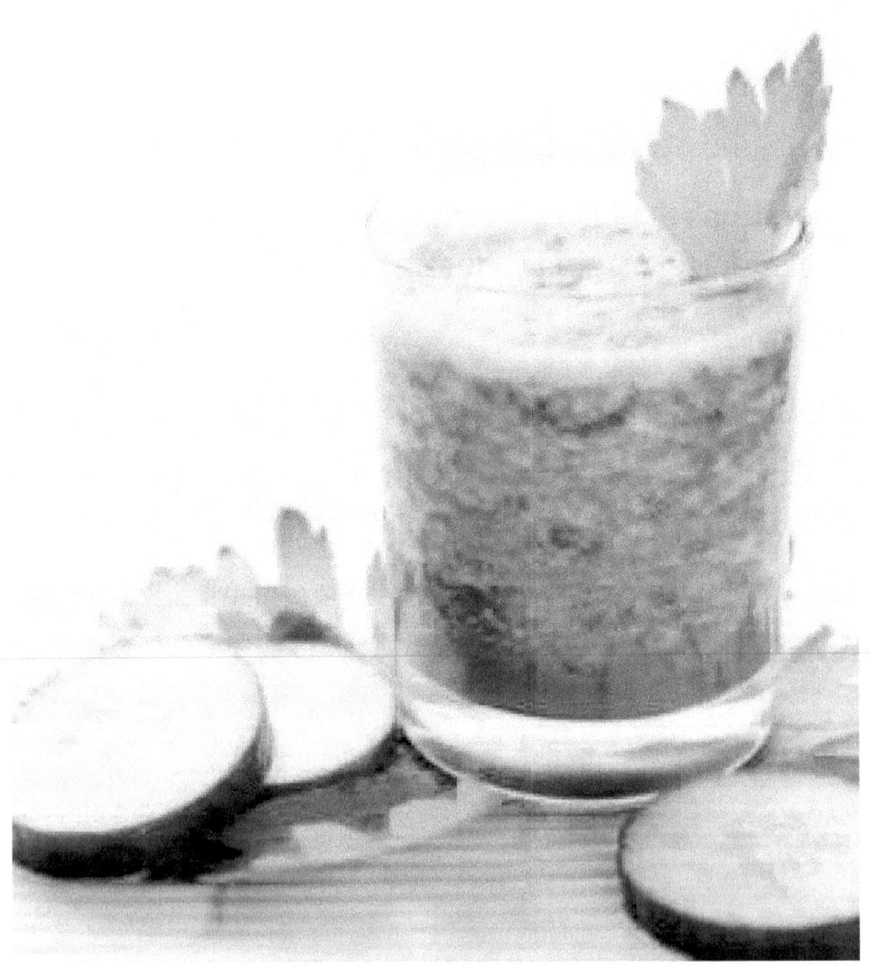

Nori Smoothie

Ingredients:

2 Bananas (The smallest one or the Burro/midsize/original banana)

Chamomile tea, ¼ cup

Nori (Sea Vegetable), ½ cup

Instructions:

1. Boil ¼ cup of water. Add ½ teaspoon of chamomile and let it steep for 10-15 minutes.

2. Strain and let it cool.

3. Cut bananas for the blender.

4. Blend all ingredients in a high-speed blender until smooth.

5. Enjoy!

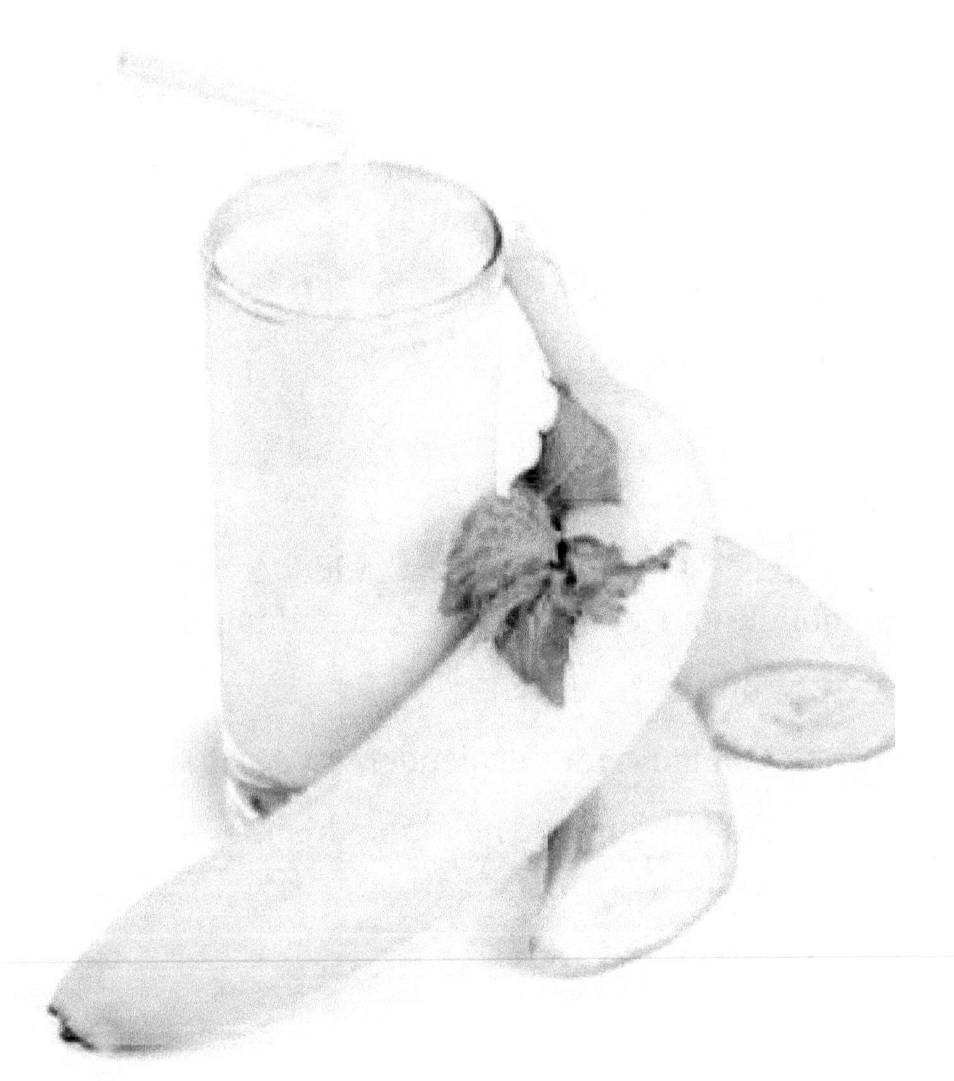

Prickly Pear Smoothie

Ingredients:

Prickly Pear (Cactus fruit), peeled, chopped, 1 cup

Date Sugar, 2 teaspoons

1 Bananas (The smallest one or the Burro/midsize/original banana)

Instructions:

1. Cut banana for the blender.

2. Blend all ingredients in a high-speed blender until smooth.

3. Enjoy!

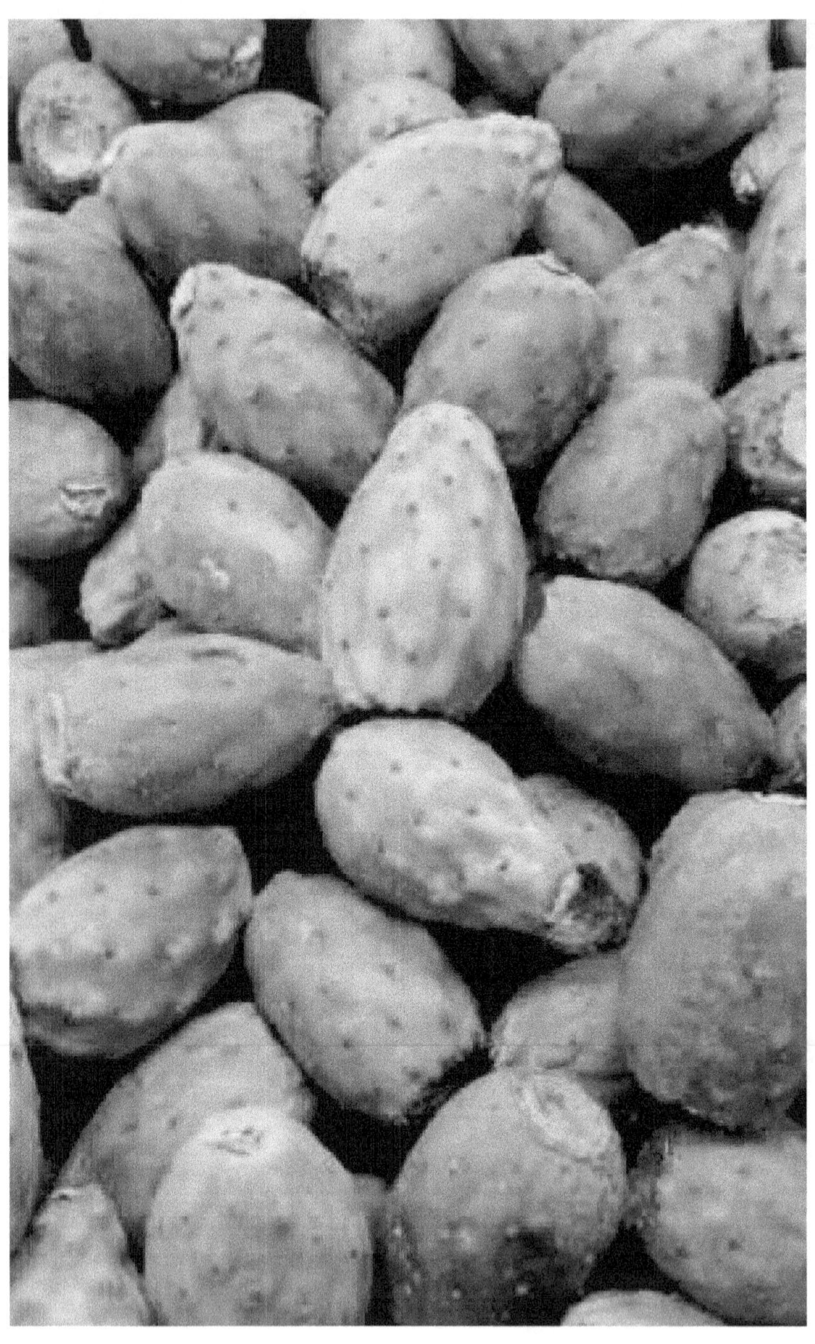

Pure Avocado Smoothie

Ingredients:

Soft Jelly Coconut Milk (or homemade walnut milk), ½ cup

Date Sugar, 3 teaspoons

1 Avocado, peeled, pitted

Instructions:

1.   Cut avocado for the blender.

2.   Blend all ingredients in a high-speed blender until smooth.

3.   Enjoy!

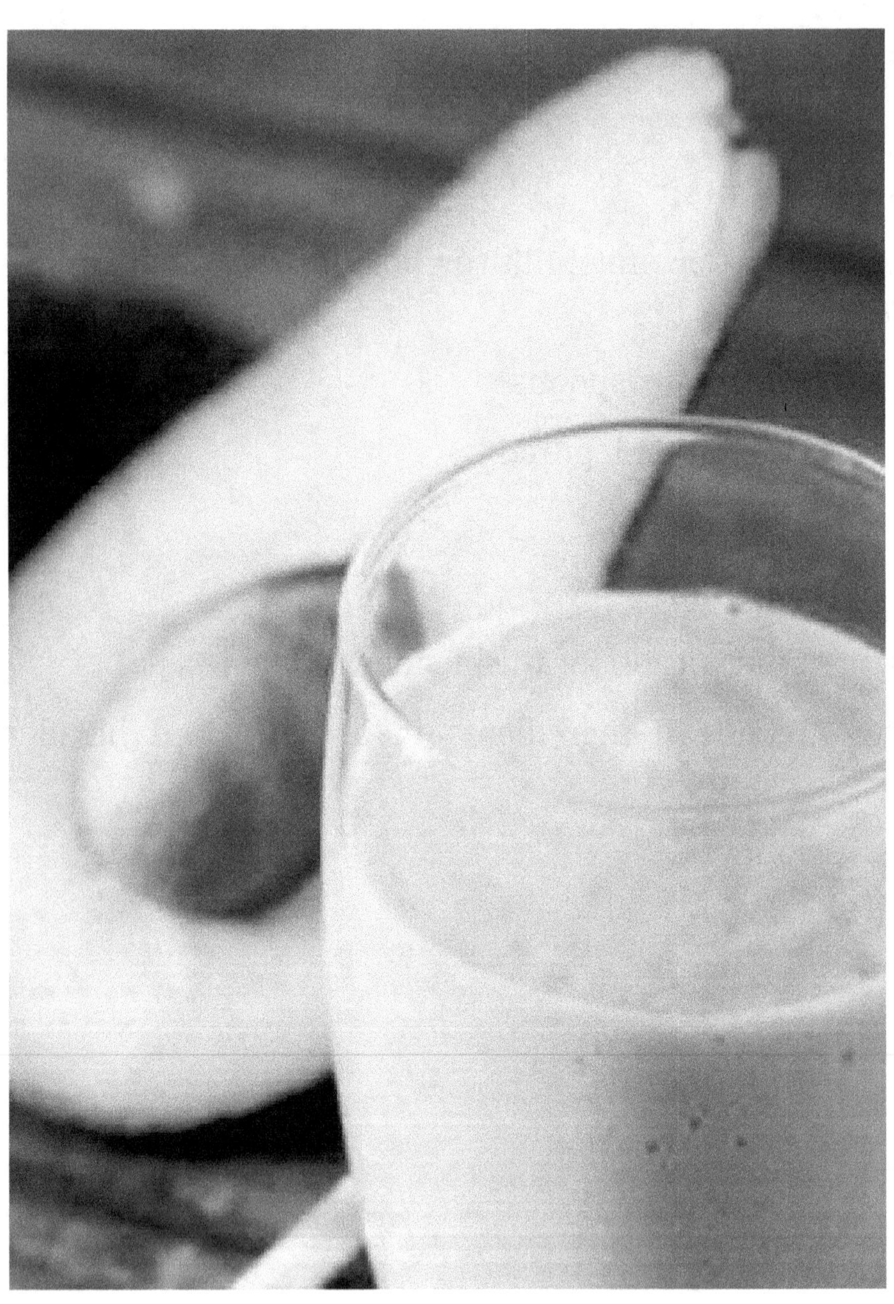

Recovery Smoothie

Ingredients:

Soft Jelly Coconut Milk (or homemade walnut milk), ¼ cup

Date Sugar, 3 teaspoons

Cherries, pitted, ½ cup

1 Bananas (The smallest one or the Burro/midsize/original banana)

Instructions:

1. Cut banana for the blender.

2. Blend all ingredients in a high-speed blender until smooth.

3. Enjoy!

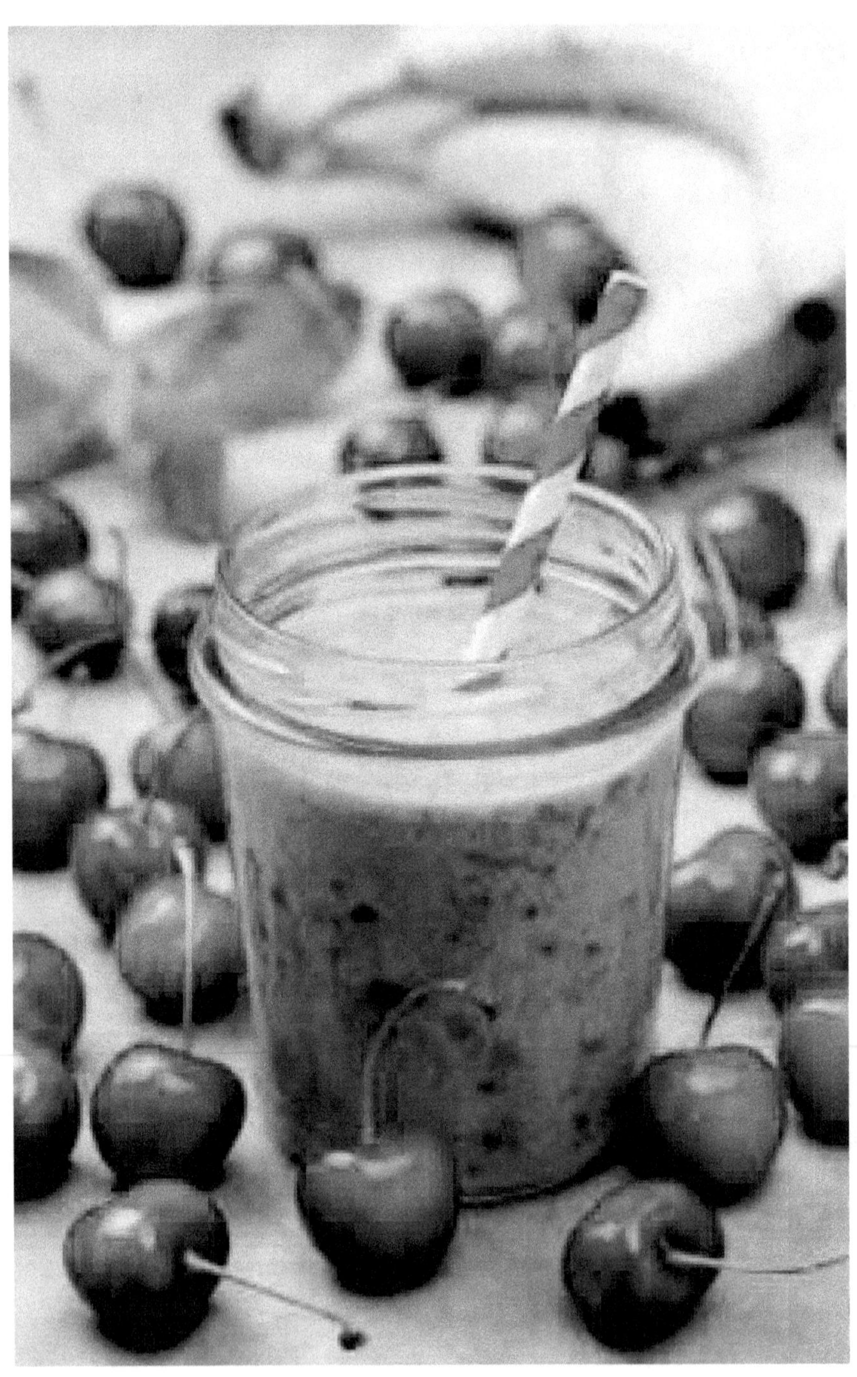

Soursops Smoothie

Ingredients:

Soft Jelly Coconut Milk (or homemade walnut milk), ½ cup

Date Sugar, 2 teaspoons

Soursops, pitted, peeled, ½ cup

Instructions:

1.   Cut soursops for the blender.

2.   Blend all ingredients in a high-speed blender until smooth.

3.   Pour the mixture into a nut milk bag.

4.   Enjoy!

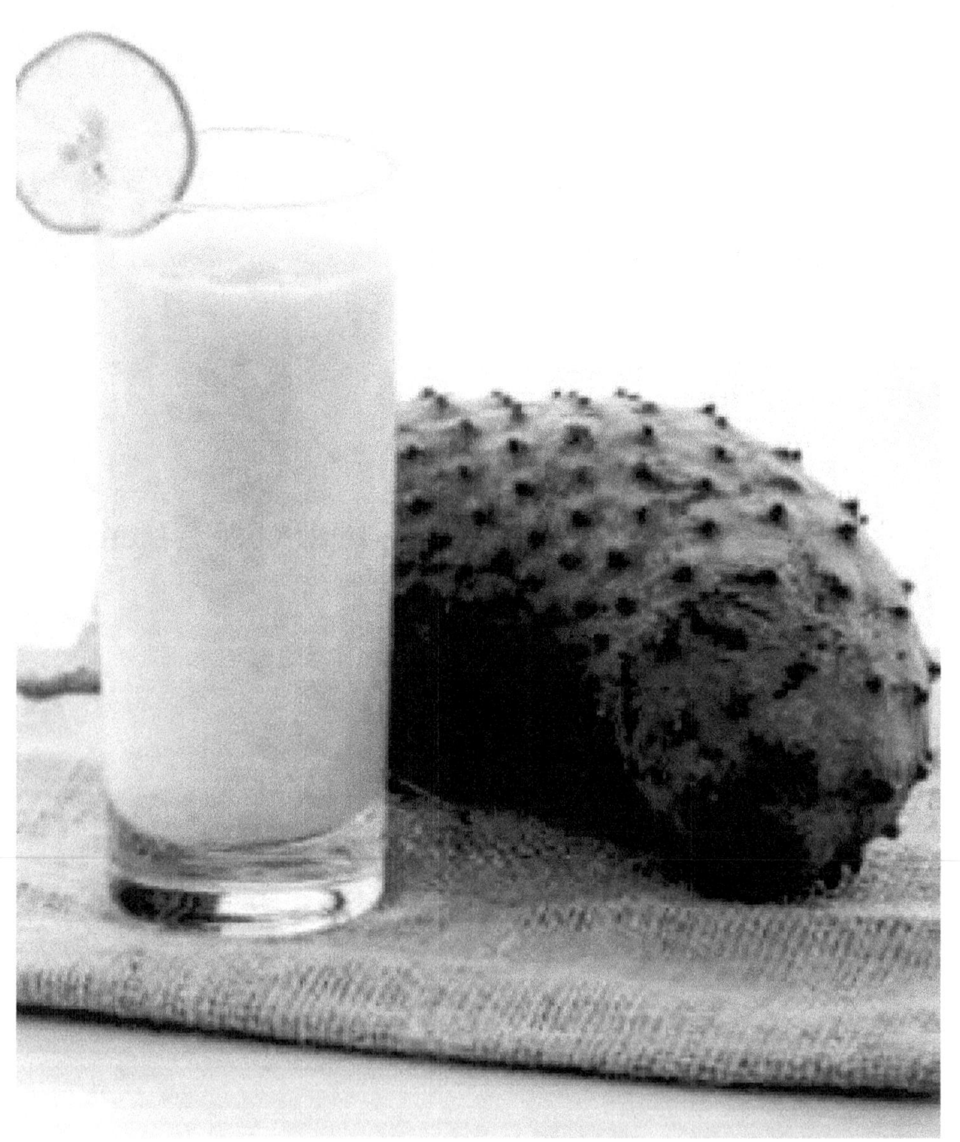

Ocean Blue Smoothie

Ingredients:

Soft Jelly Coconut Milk (or homemade walnut milk), ¼ cup

Date Sugar, 2 teaspoons

2 Bananas (The smallest one or the Burro/midsizc/original banana)

Blueberries, ¼ cup

Blackberries, ¼ cup

Instructions:

1. Cut bananas for the blender.

2. Blend all ingredients in a high-speed blender until creamy.

3. Enjoy!

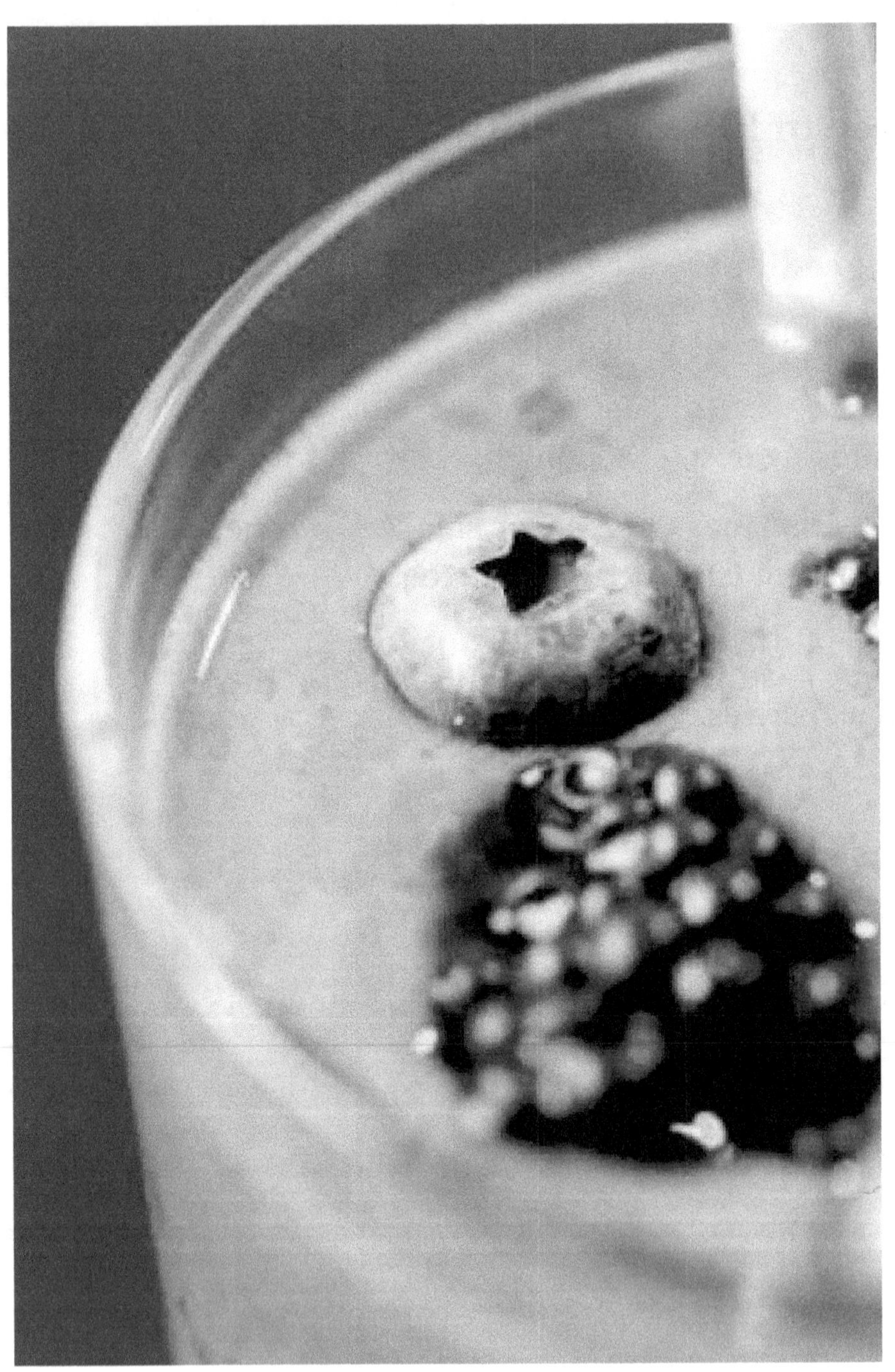

Tomato Smoothie

Ingredients:

Tomato (Cherry and plum only), 1 cup

Pure Sea Salt, To taste

Basil, 3 leaves

Instructions:

1.	Cut tomatoes for the blender.

2.	Blend all ingredients in a high-speed blender until smooth.

3.	Pour the mixture into a nut milk bag.

4.	Enjoy!

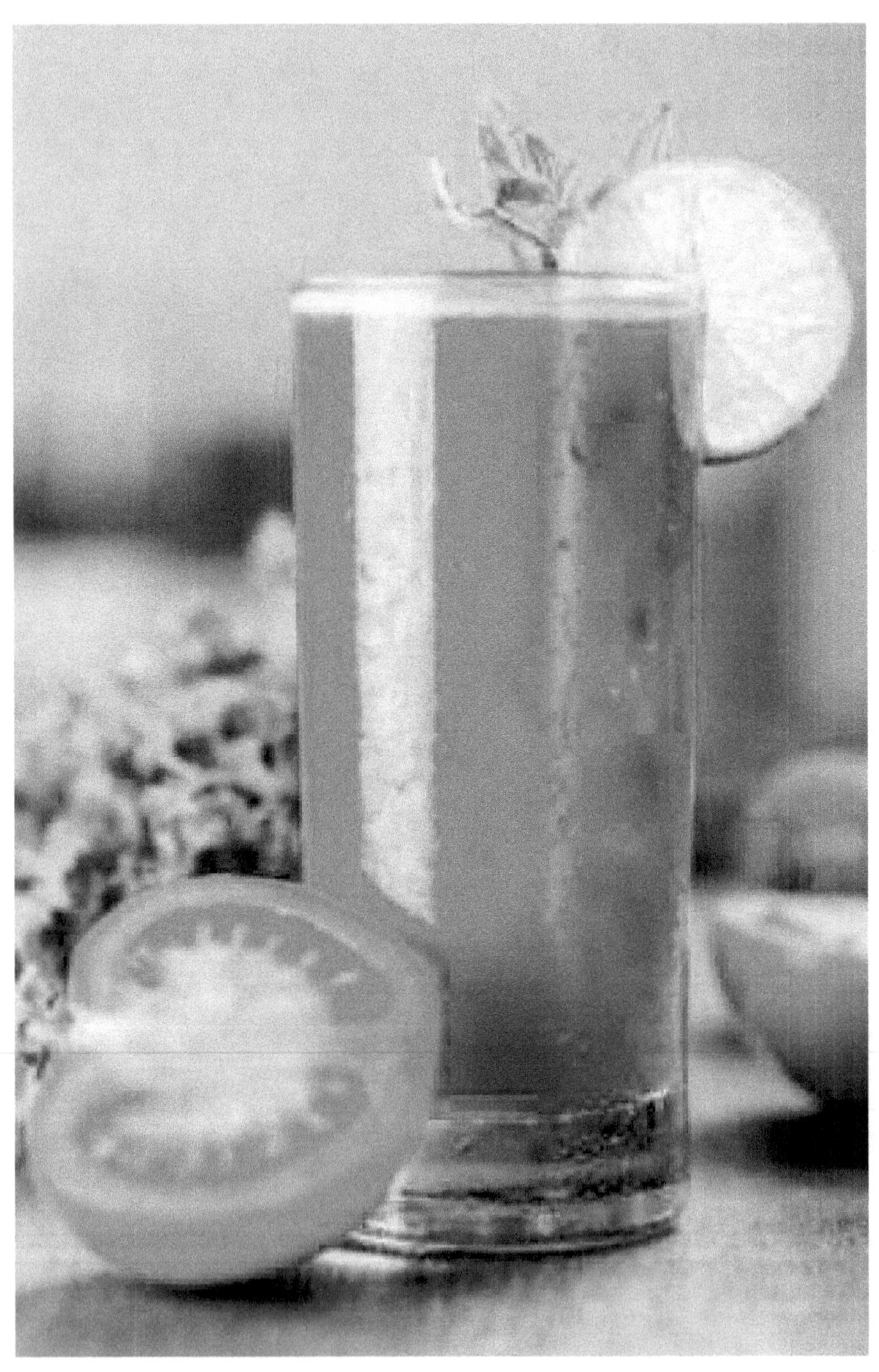

Berryland Smoothie

Ingredients:

Soft Jelly Coconut Milk (or homemade walnut milk), ½ cup

Date Sugar, 3 teaspoons

Blueberries, ¼ cup

Blackberries, ¼ cup

Raspberries, ¼ cup

Strawberries, ¼ cup

Currants, ¼ cup

Instructions:

1. Blend all ingredients in a high-speed blender until smooth.

2. Enjoy!

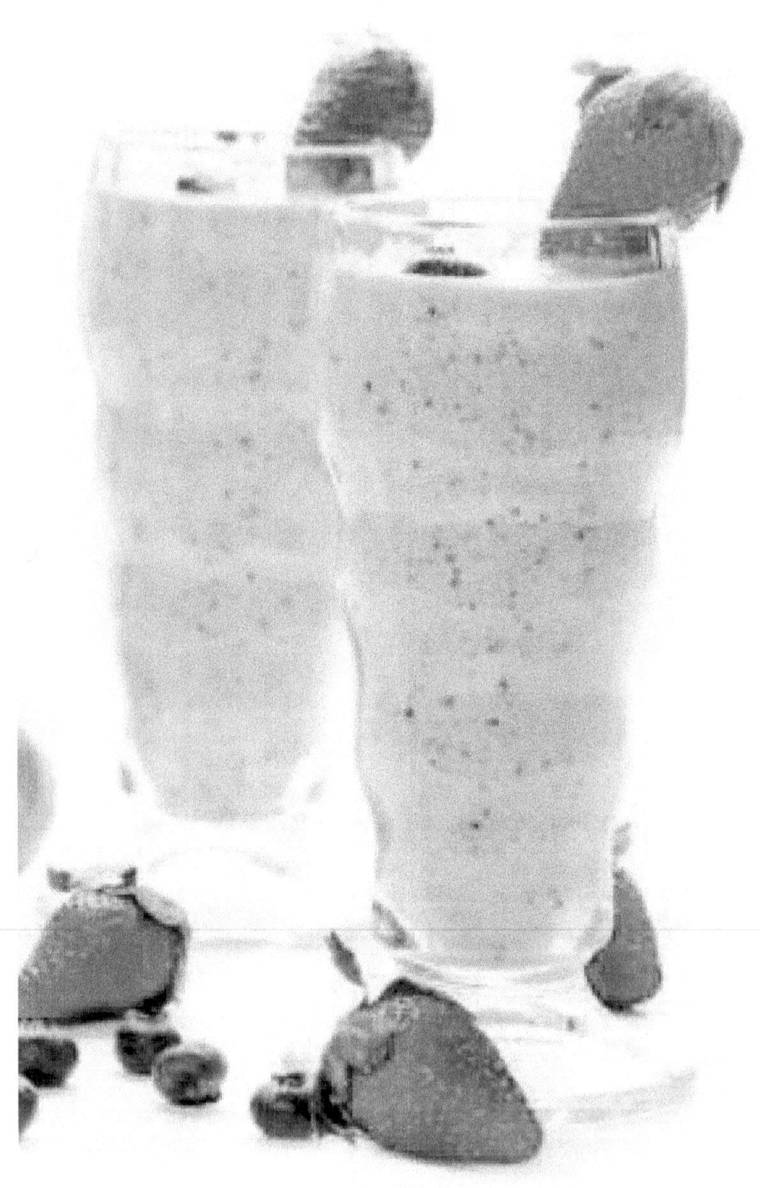

Green Tonic Smoothie

Ingredients:

Izote (Cactus leaf), ½ cup

Melons (Seeded), 6 oz (170 g)

Lettuce (All, except Iceberg), chopped, ¼ cup

Date Sugar, 2 teaspoons

Instructions:

1.   Cut izote and melon for the blender.

2.   Blend all ingredients in a high-speed blender until smooth.

3.   Enjoy!

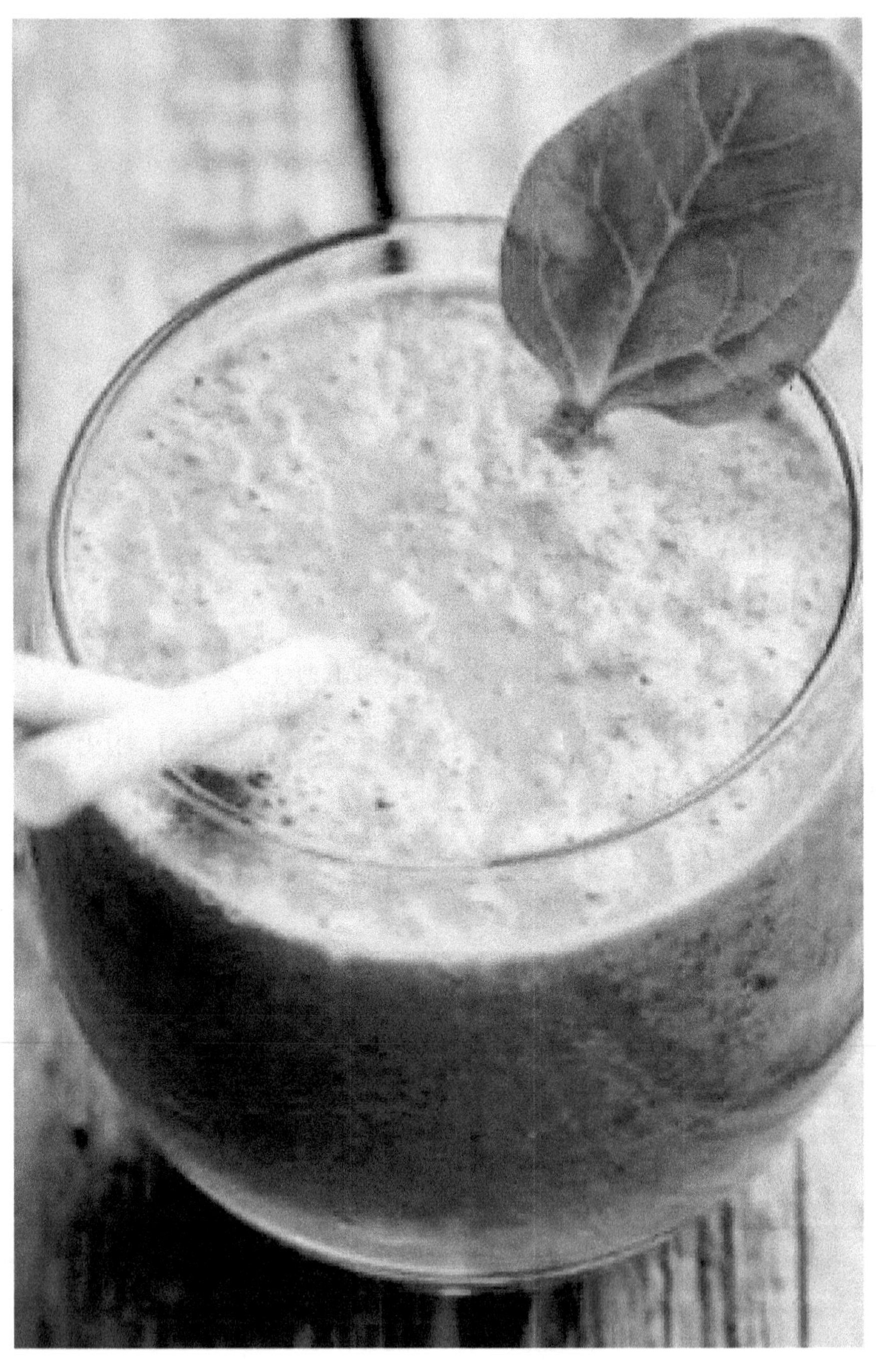

Hearty Smoothie

Ingredients:

½ Avocado, peeled, pitted

Date Sugar, 2 teaspoons

1 Apples, pitted

Grapes (Seeded), ¼ cup

1 Bananas (The smallest one or the Burro/midsize/original banana)

Instructions:

1. Cut banana, apple, and avocado for the blender.

2. Blend all ingredients in a high-speed blender until smooth.

3. Enjoy!

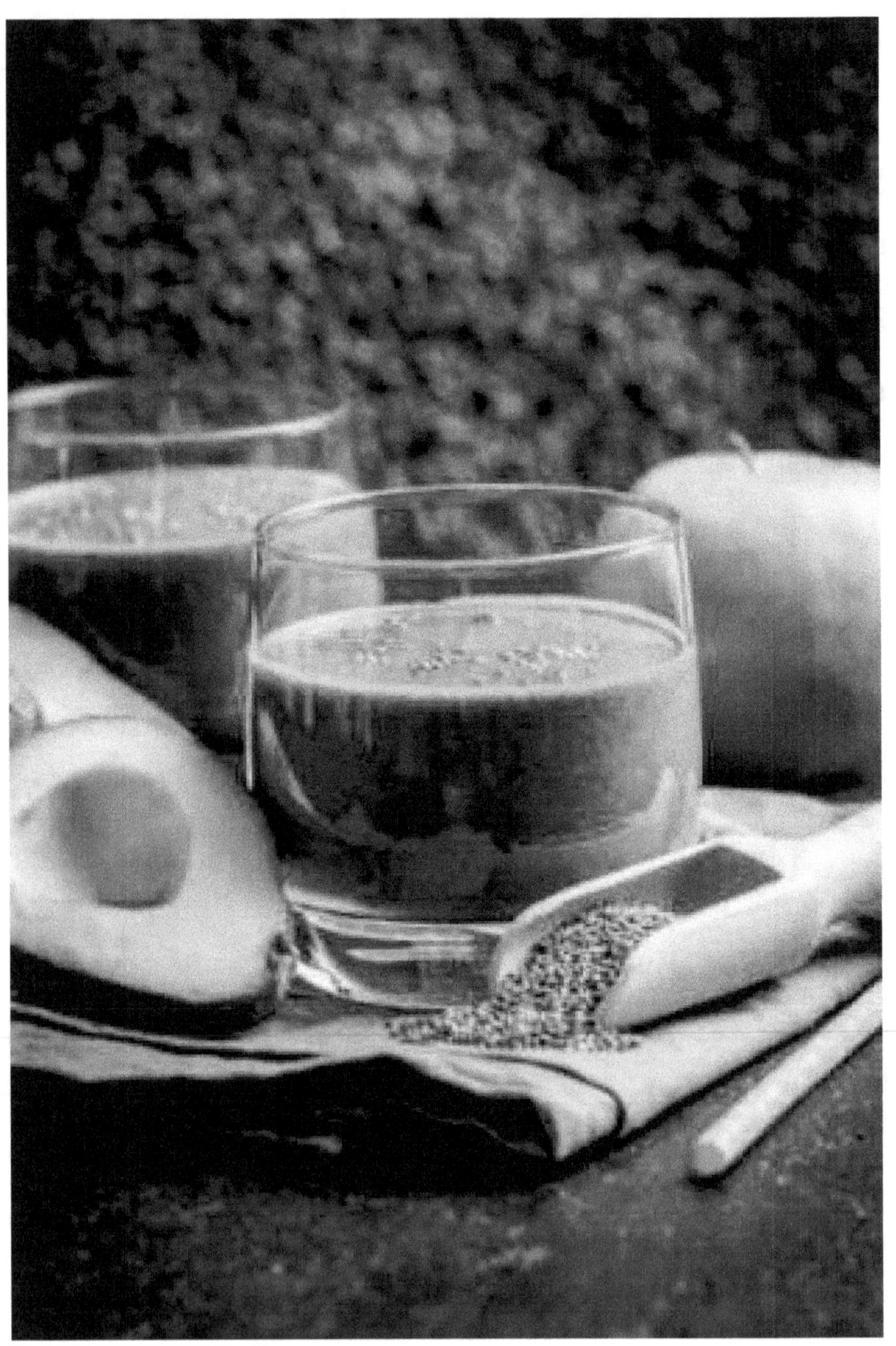

Dulse Smoothie

Ingredients:

1 Bananas (The smallest one or the Burro/midsize/original banana)

Date Sugar, 2 teaspoons

Blueberries, ¼ cup

Dulse (Sea Vegetable), ½ cup

Instructions:

1.   Cut banana for the blender.

2.   Blend all ingredients in a high-speed blender until smooth.

3.   Enjoy!

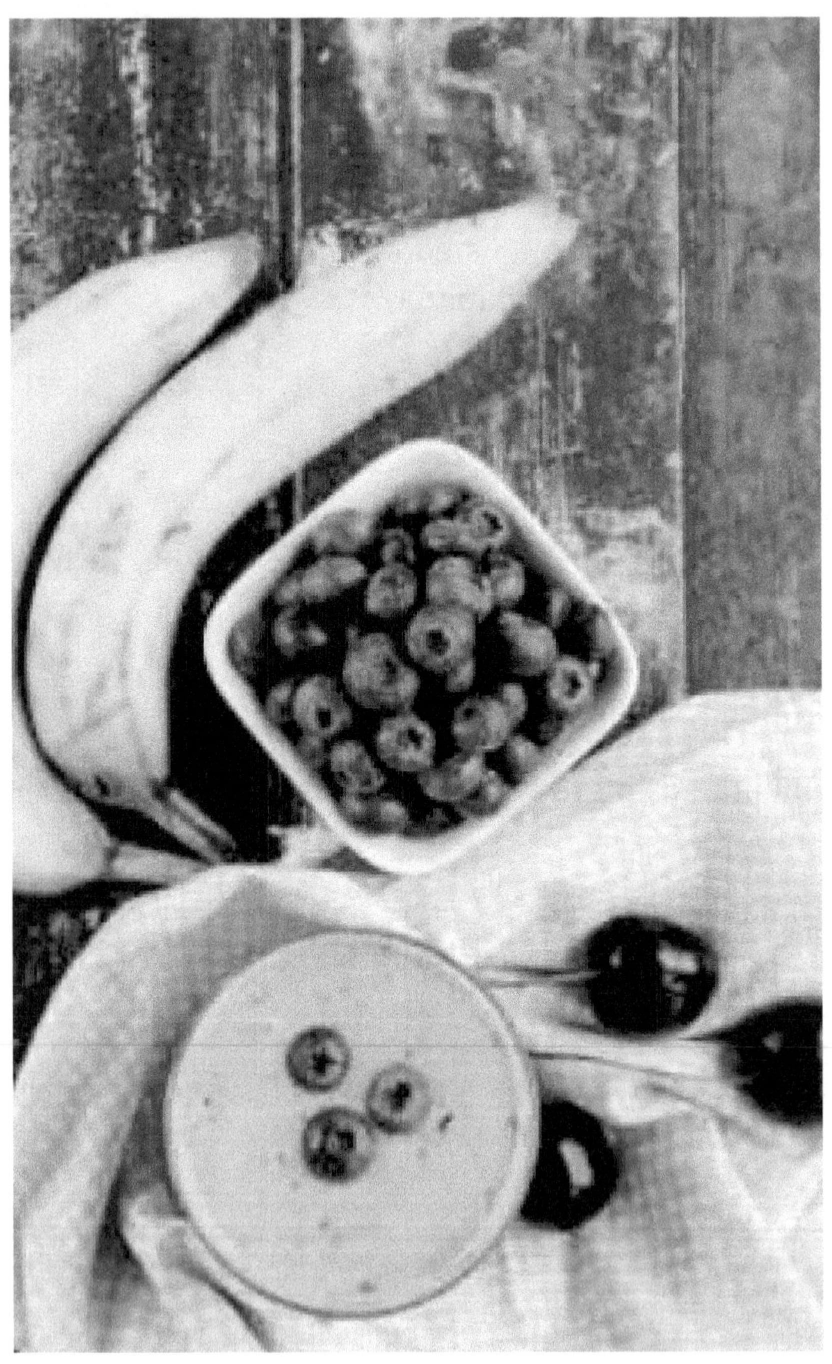

Anti-Cholesterol Smoothie

Ingredients:

Kale, chopped, ¾ cup

Date Sugar, 2 teaspoons

1 Bananas (The smallest one or the Burro/midsize/original banana)

Instructions:

1. Cut banana for the blender.

2. Blend all ingredients in a high-speed blender until smooth.

3. Enjoy!

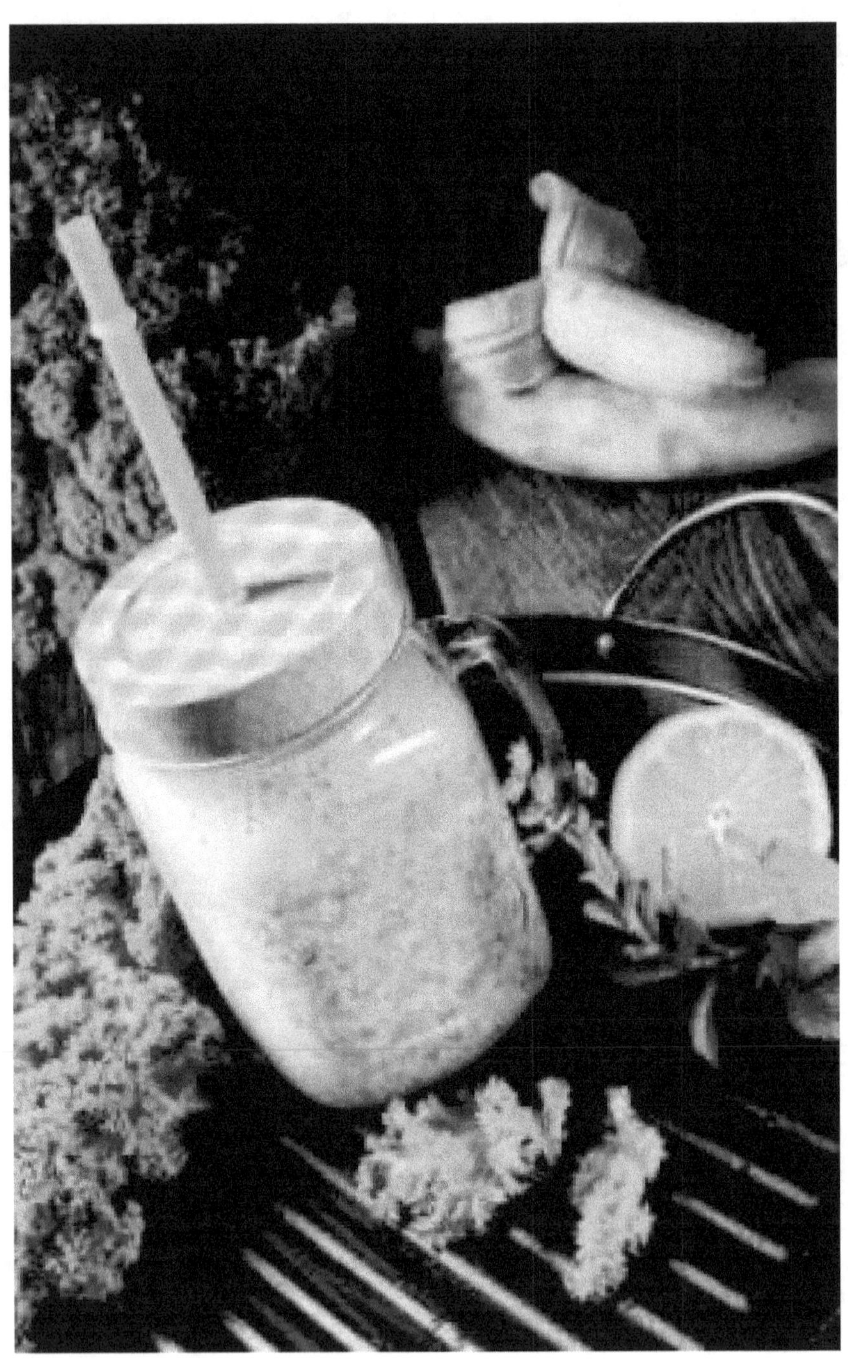

Anti-Inflammation Smoothie

Ingredients:

Lettuce (All, except Iceberg), chopped, ½ cup

1 Apples, pitted

Date Sugar, 2 teaspoons

Ginger, grated, ¼ teaspoons

1 Bananas (The smallest one or the Burro/midsize/original banana)

Instructions:

1. Cut banana and apple for the blender.

2. Blend all ingredients in a high-speed blender until smooth.

3. Enjoy!

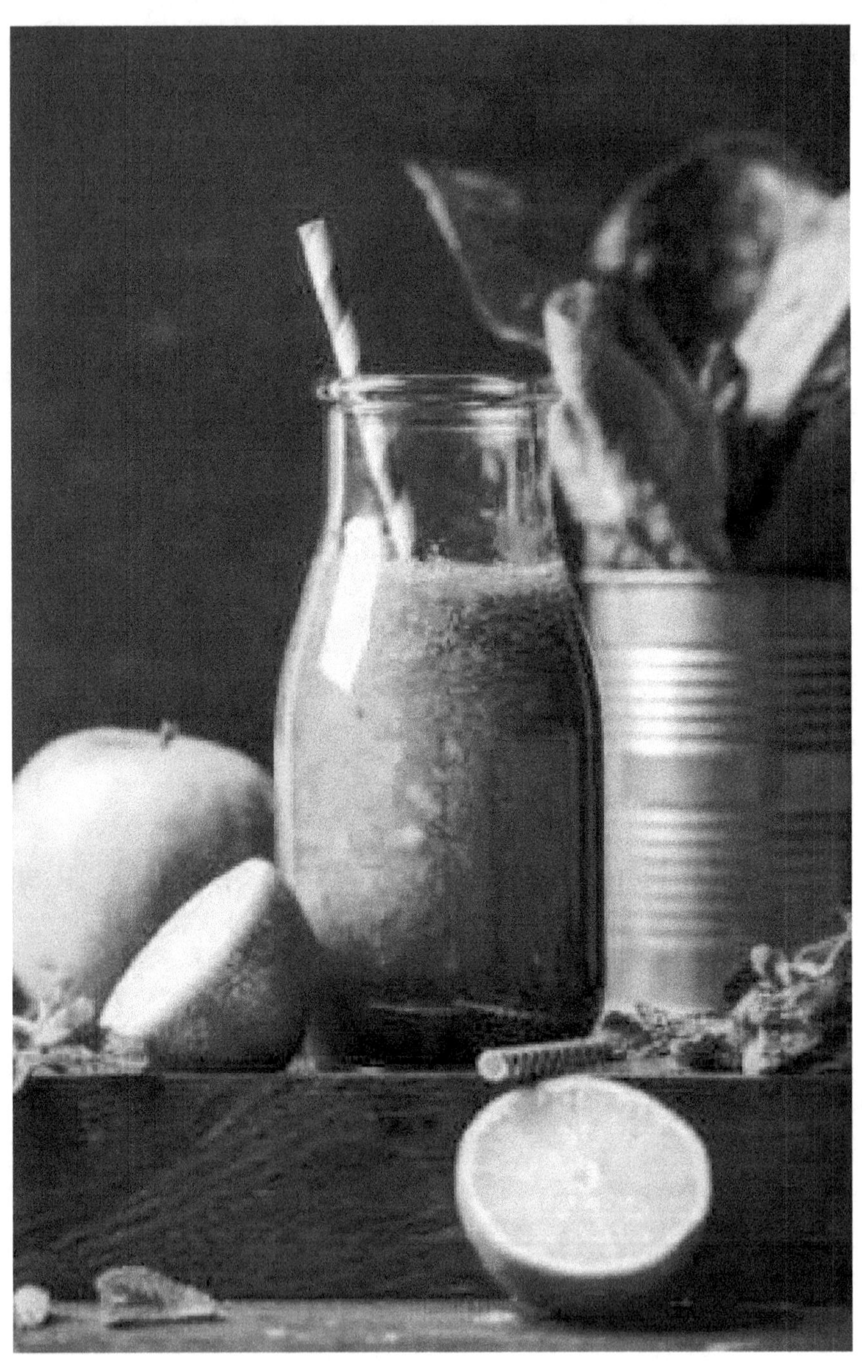

Heart-Healthy Smoothie

Ingredients:

½ Avocado, peeled, pitted

Date Sugar, 2 teaspoons

Lime juice, 1 teaspoon

2 Apples, pitted

1 Bananas (The smallest one or the Burro/midsize/original banana)

Instructions:

1. Cut banana, apples, and avocado for the blender.

2. Blend all ingredients in a high-speed blender until smooth.

3. Enjoy!

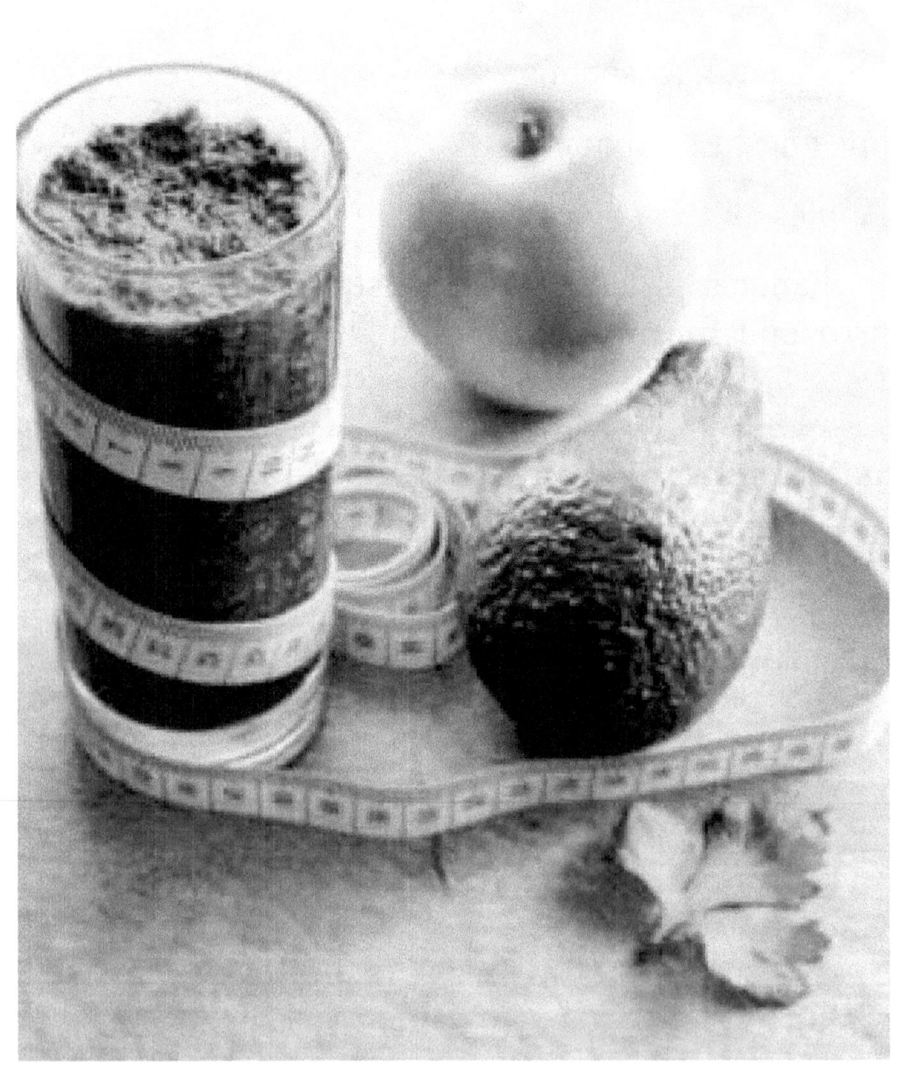

Purslane Smoothie

Ingredients:

Date Sugar, 2 teaspoons

Purslane (Verdolaga), chopped, 1 cup

Ginger, grated, ¼ teaspoons

Instructions:

1. Blend all ingredients in a high-speed blender until smooth.

2. Pour the mixture into a nut milk bag.

3. Enjoy!

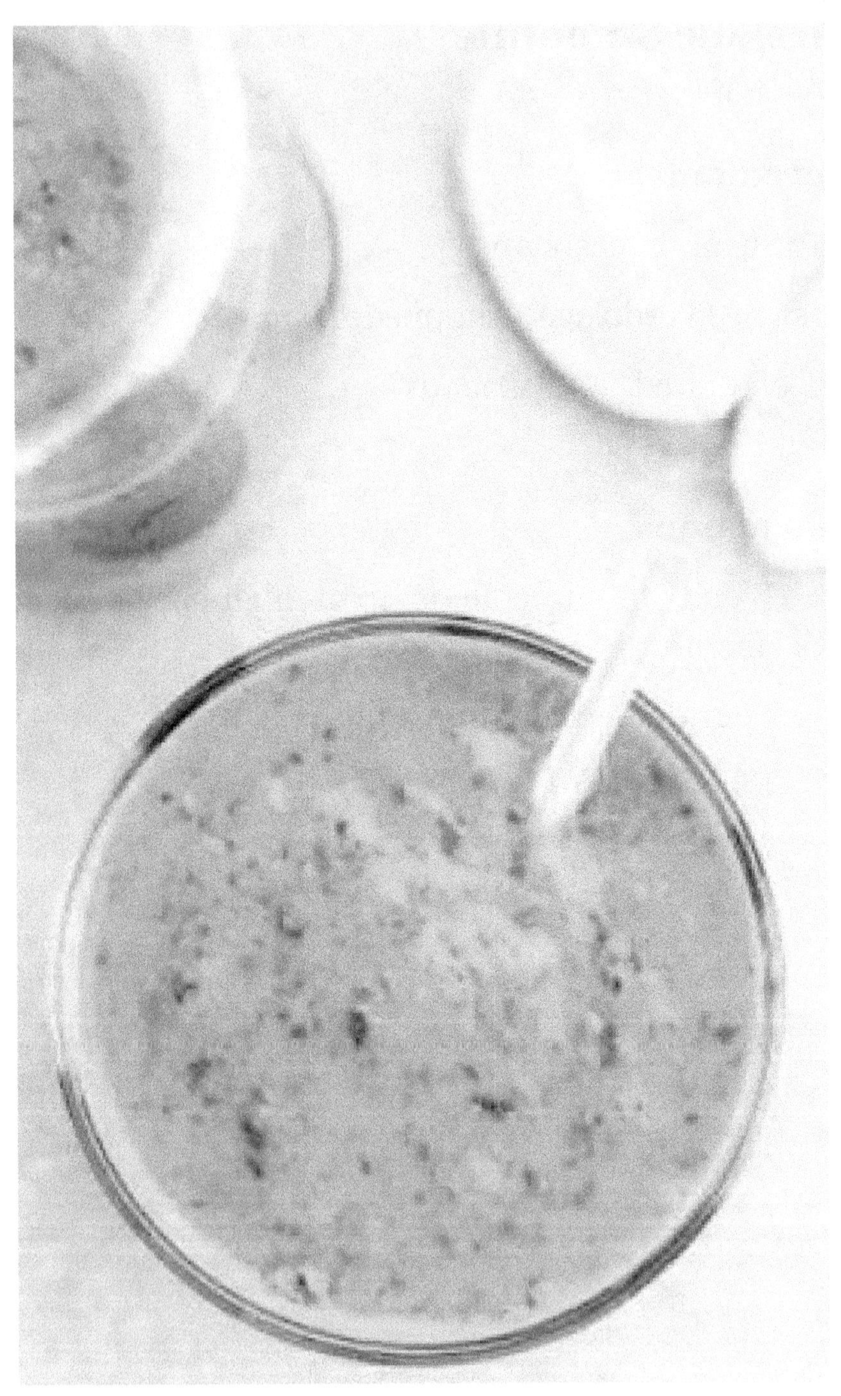

Anti-Allergy Smoothie

Ingredients:

¼ cup Soft Jelly Coconut Milk (or homemade walnut milk)

4 Peaches, pitted

Instructions:

1.   Blend all ingredients in a high-speed blender until smooth.

2.   Enjoy!

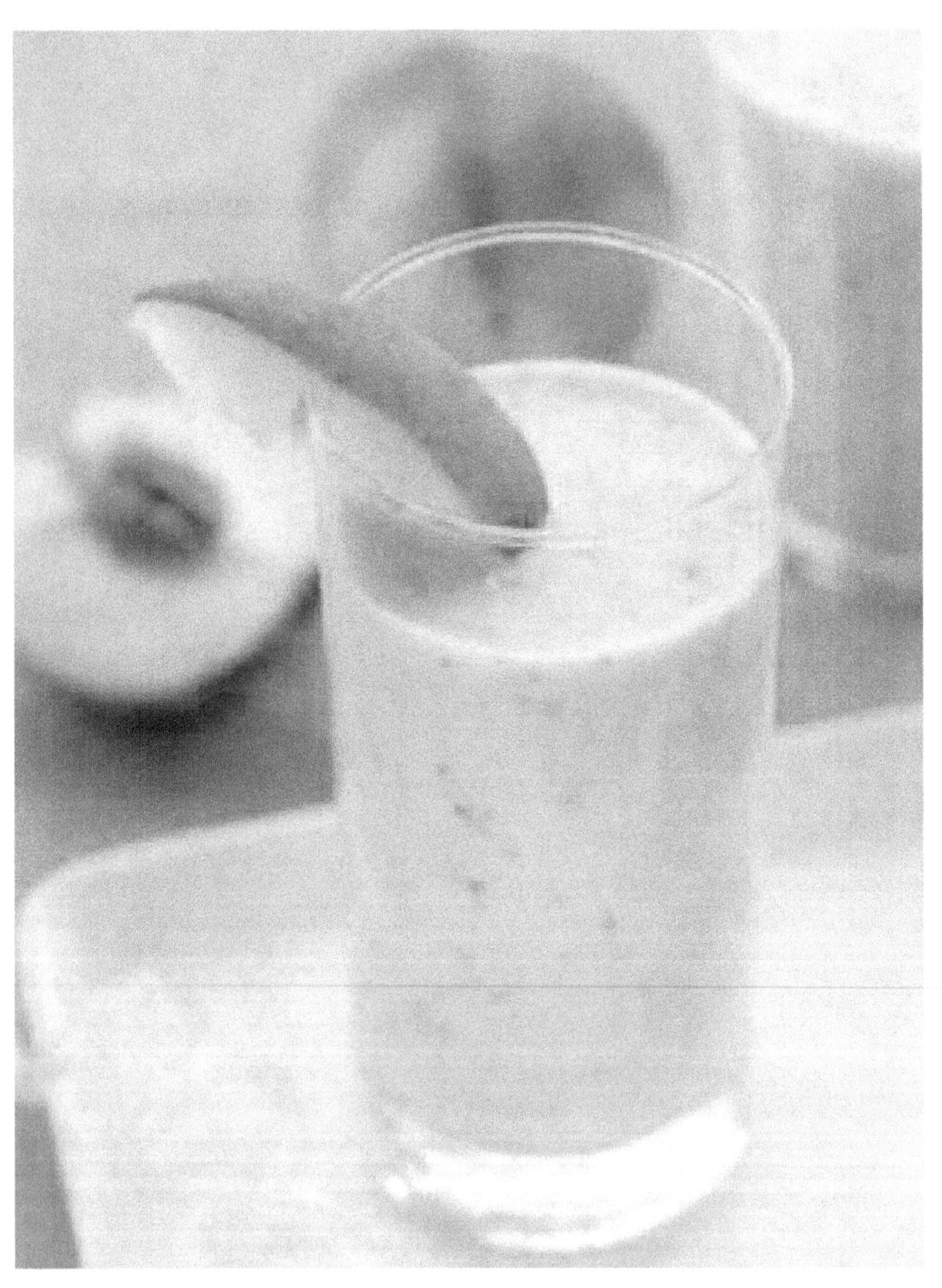

Three-Berry Smoothie

Ingredients:

Blueberries, 1/3 cup

Raspberries, 1/3 cup

Strawberries, 1/3 cup

Ginger, grated, ¼ teaspoons

Instructions:

1.   Blend all ingredients in a high-speed blender until smooth.

2.   Enjoy!

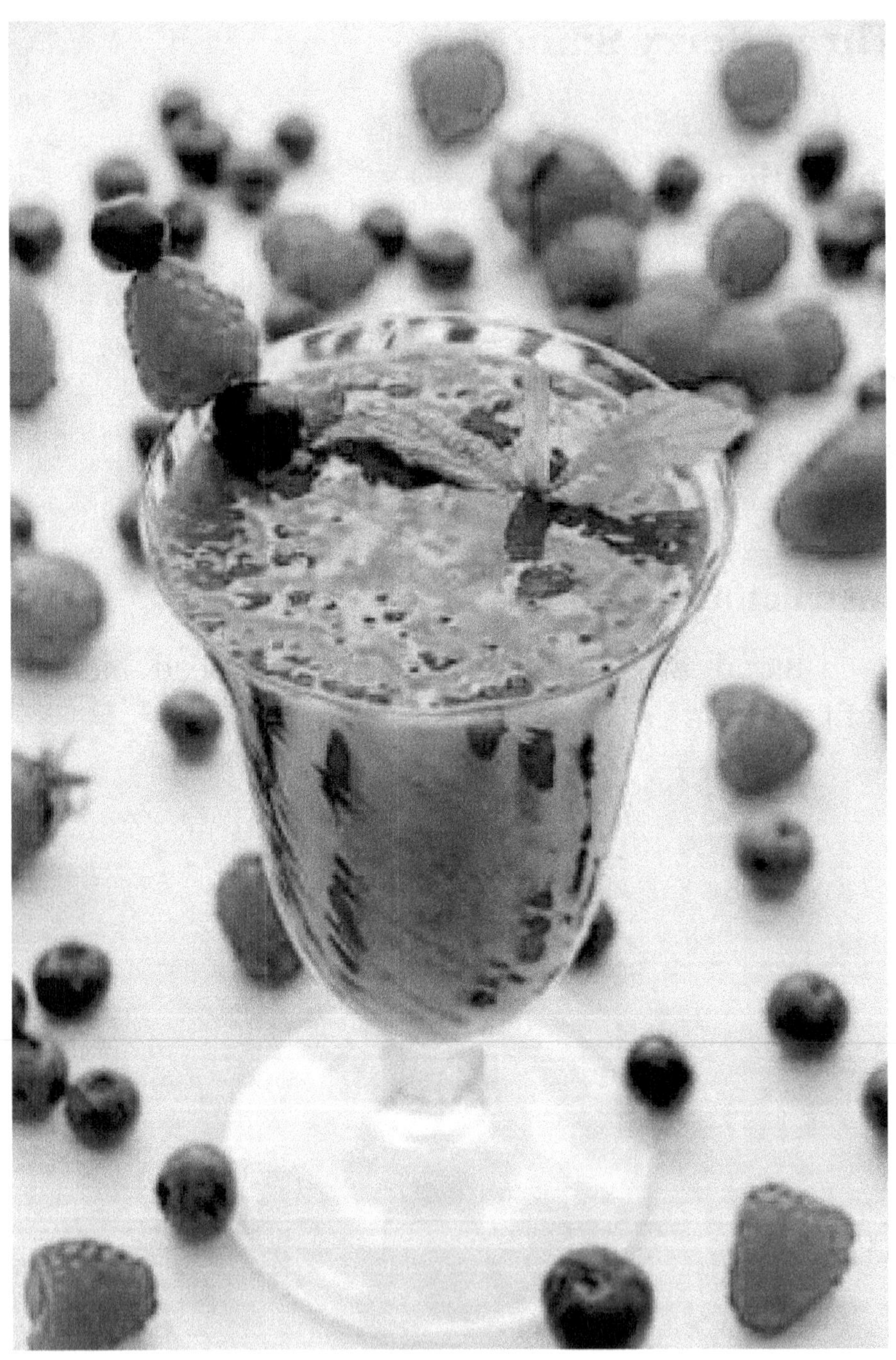

Ice Cream Smoothie

Ingredients:

Ice, cubed, ½ cup

Date Sugar, 2 teaspoons

Soft Jelly Coconut Pulp, shredded, From 1 coconut

1 Bananas (The smallest one or the Burro/midsize/original banana)

Instructions:

1. Cut banana for the blender.

2. Blend all ingredients except for ice in a high-speed blender until creamy.

3. Add ice and blend until smooth.

4. Place smoothie into the freezer for 30 minutes.

5. Enjoy!

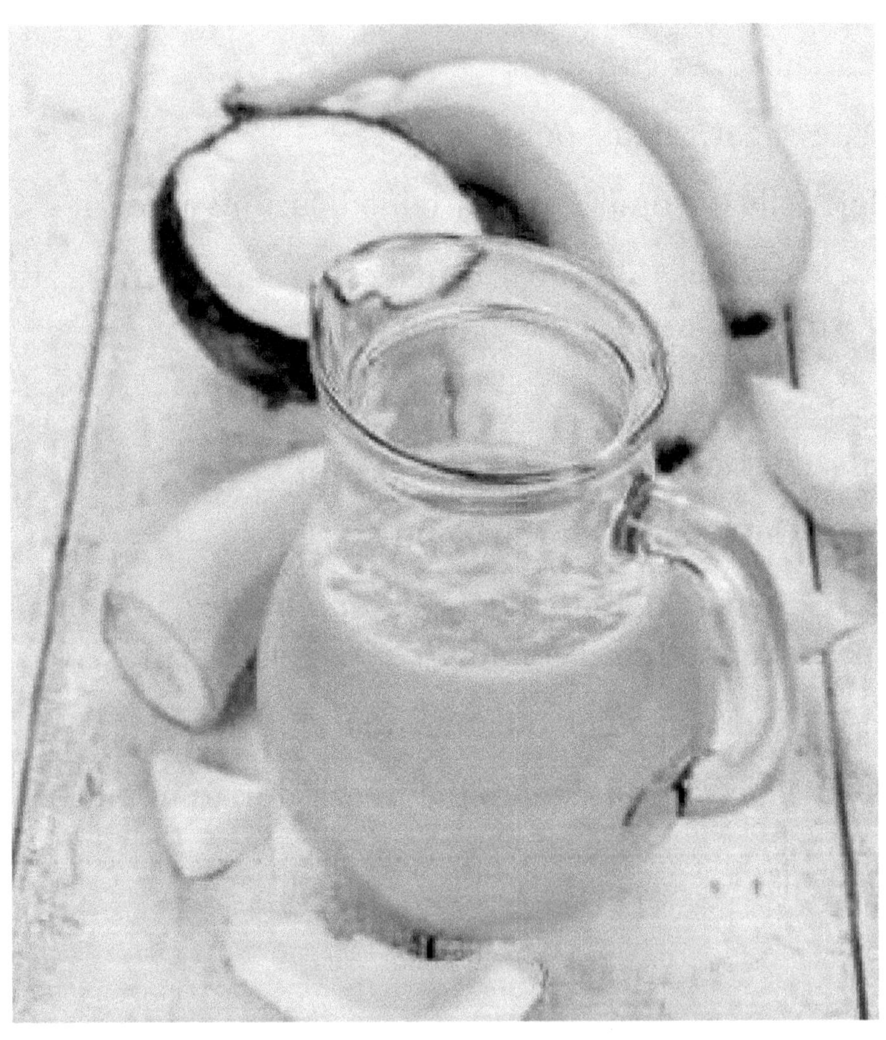

Lettuce Smoothie

Ingredients:

Fennel tea, ½ cup

Lettuce (All, except Iceberg), chopped, ½ cup

Date Sugar, 2 teaspoons

Instructions:

1.   Boil ½ cup of water. Add ½ teaspoon of fennel and let it steep for 10-15 minutes.

2.   Strain and let it cool.

3.   Blend all ingredients in a high-speed blender until smooth.

4.   Enjoy!

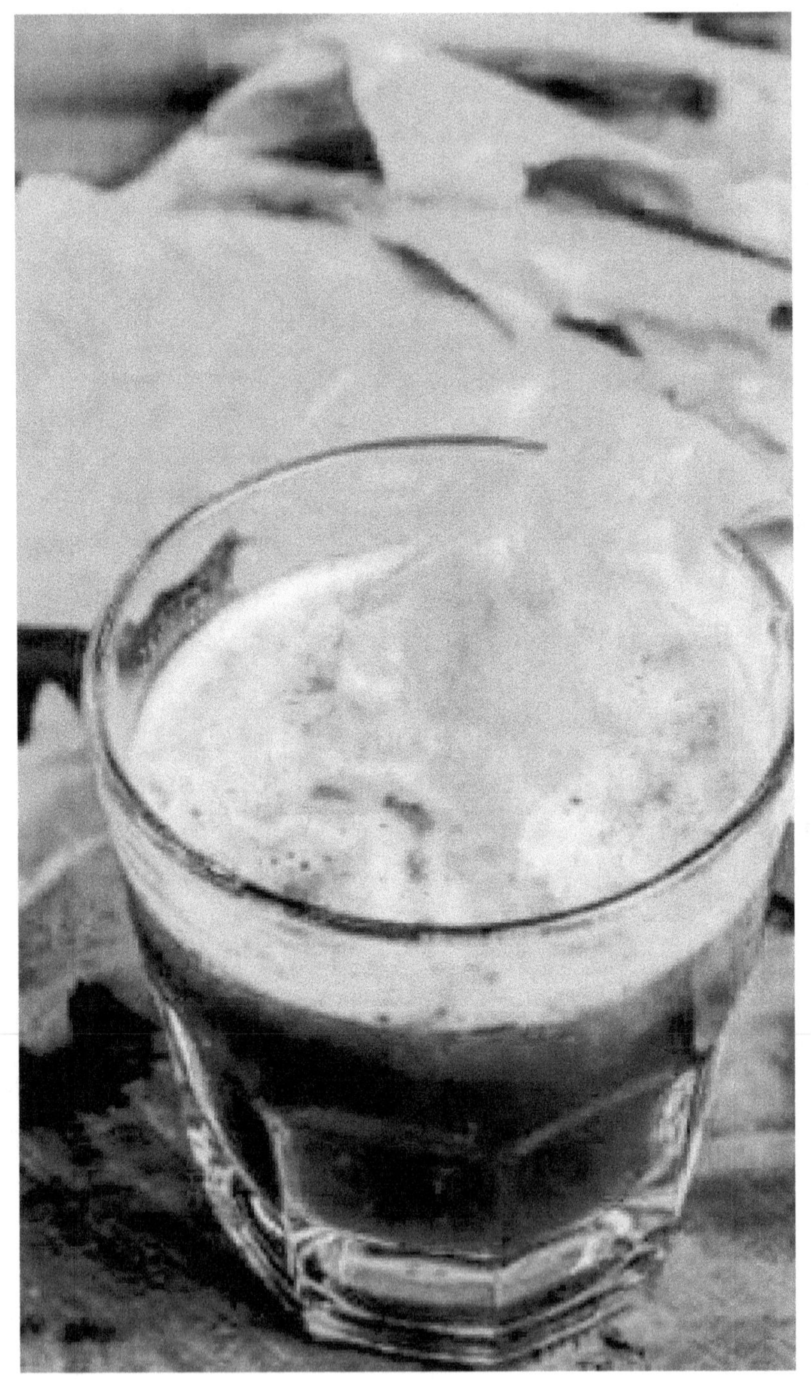

Aid Digestion Smoothie

Ingredients:

2 Peaches, pitted

Strawberries, ½ cup

Ginger, grated, ¼ teaspoons

Instructions:

1.   Cut peaches for the blender.

2.   Blend all ingredients in a high-speed blender until smooth.

3.   Enjoy!

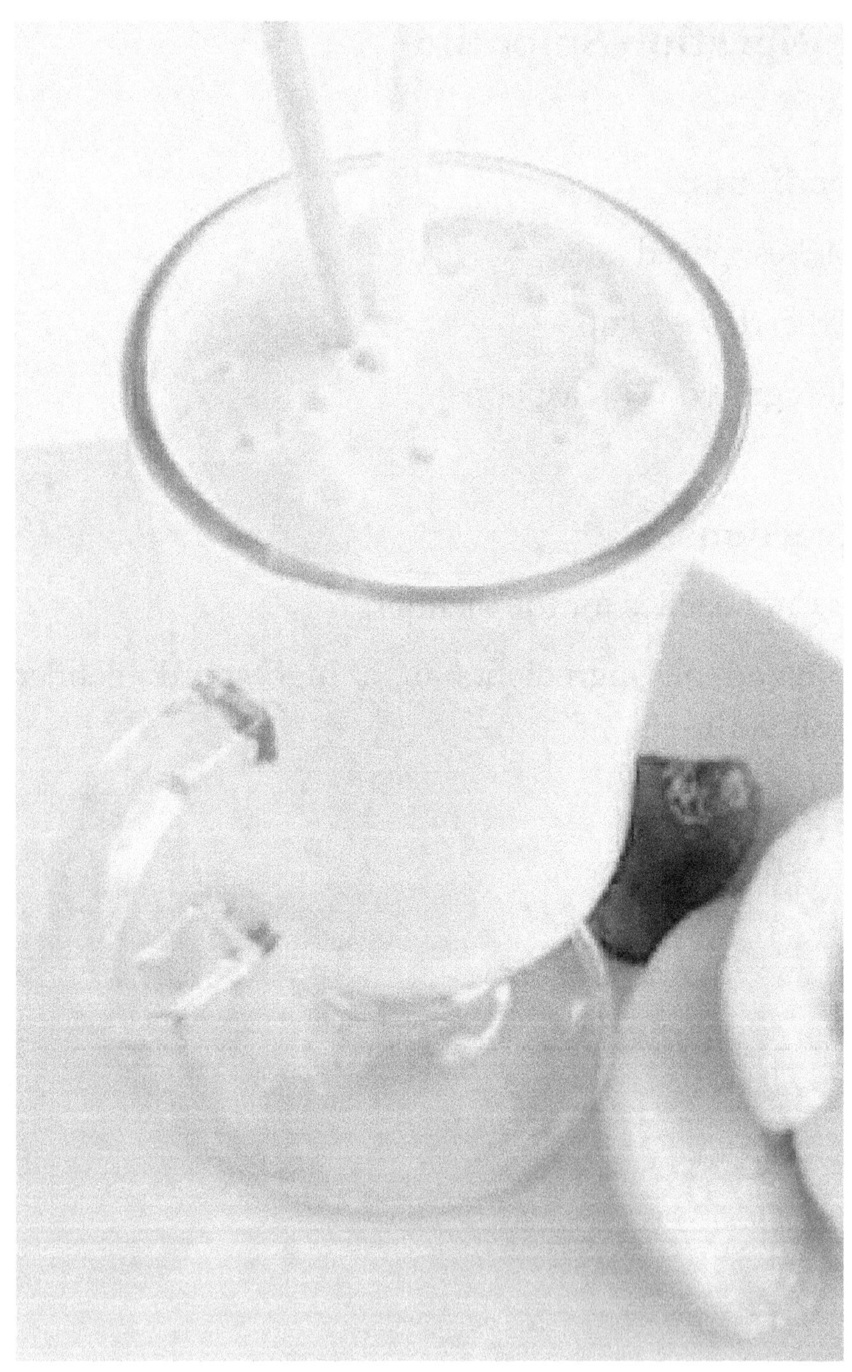

One-Third Smoothie

Ingredients:

Date Sugar, 2 teaspoons

Blueberries, 1/3 cup

Blackberries, 1/3 cup

Currants, 1/3 cup

Instructions:

1.   Blend all ingredients in a high-speed blender until smooth.

2.   Enjoy!

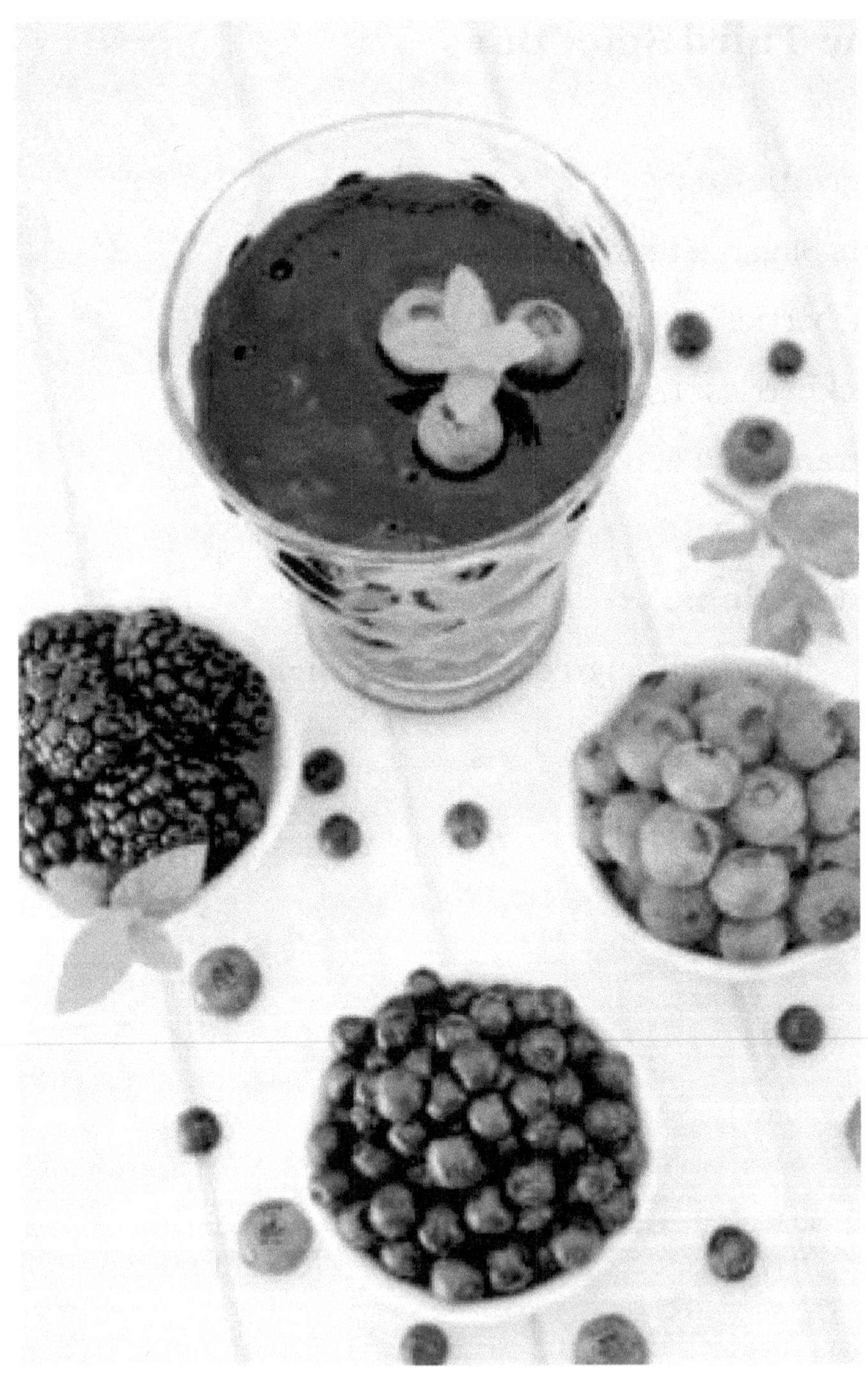

Squash Smoothie

Ingredients:

Squash, cubed, 1 cup

Date Sugar, 2 teaspoons

Instructions:

1.   Blend all ingredients in a high-speed blender until smooth.

2.   Enjoy!

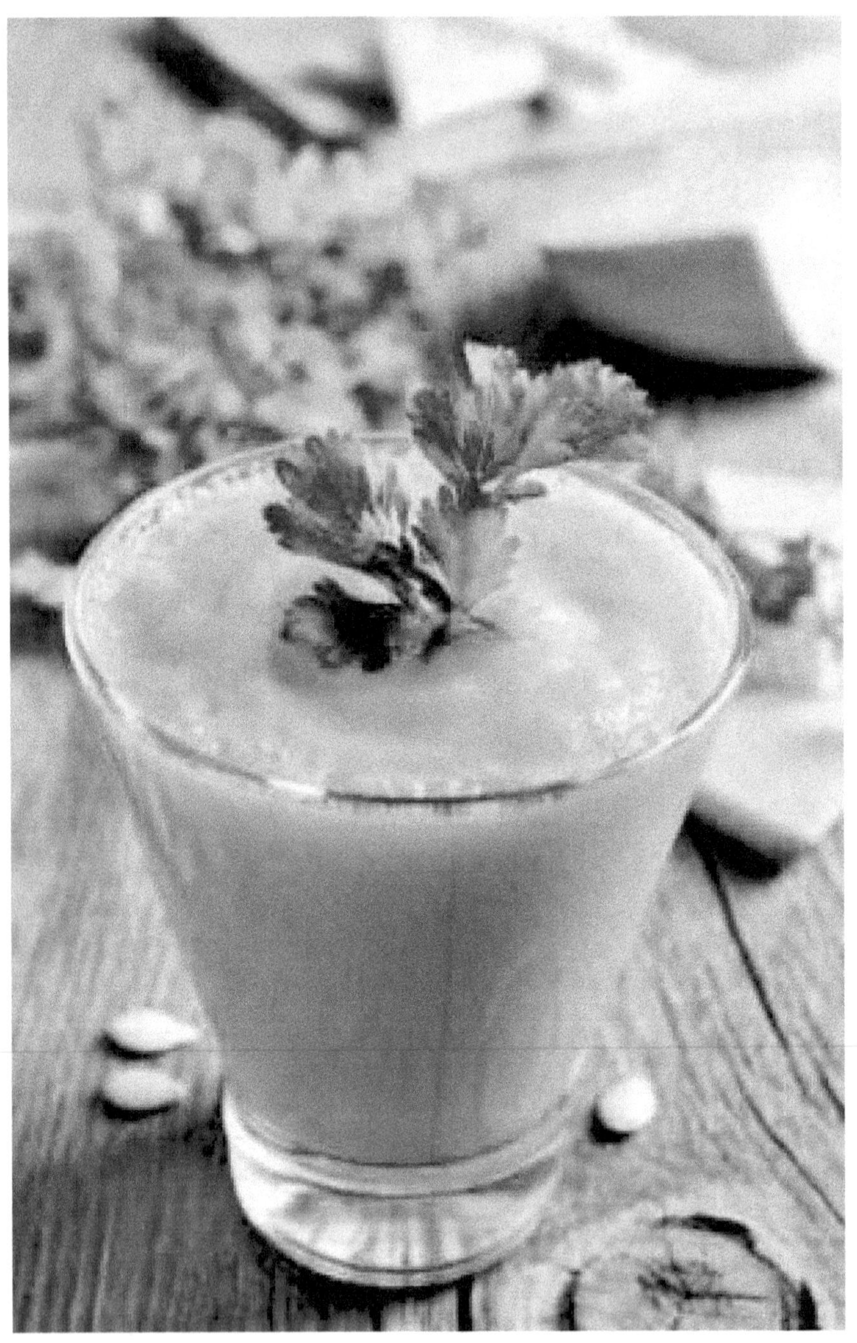

Nutty Date Smoothie

Ingredients:

Soft Jelly Coconut Milk (or homemade walnut milk), ½ cup

Dates, pitted, ¼ cup

Brazil Nuts or Walnuts, ¼ cup

1 Bananas (The smallest one or the Burro/midsize/original banana)

Instructions:

1. Cut banana for the blender.

2. Blend all ingredients in a high-speed blender until smooth.

3. Enjoy!

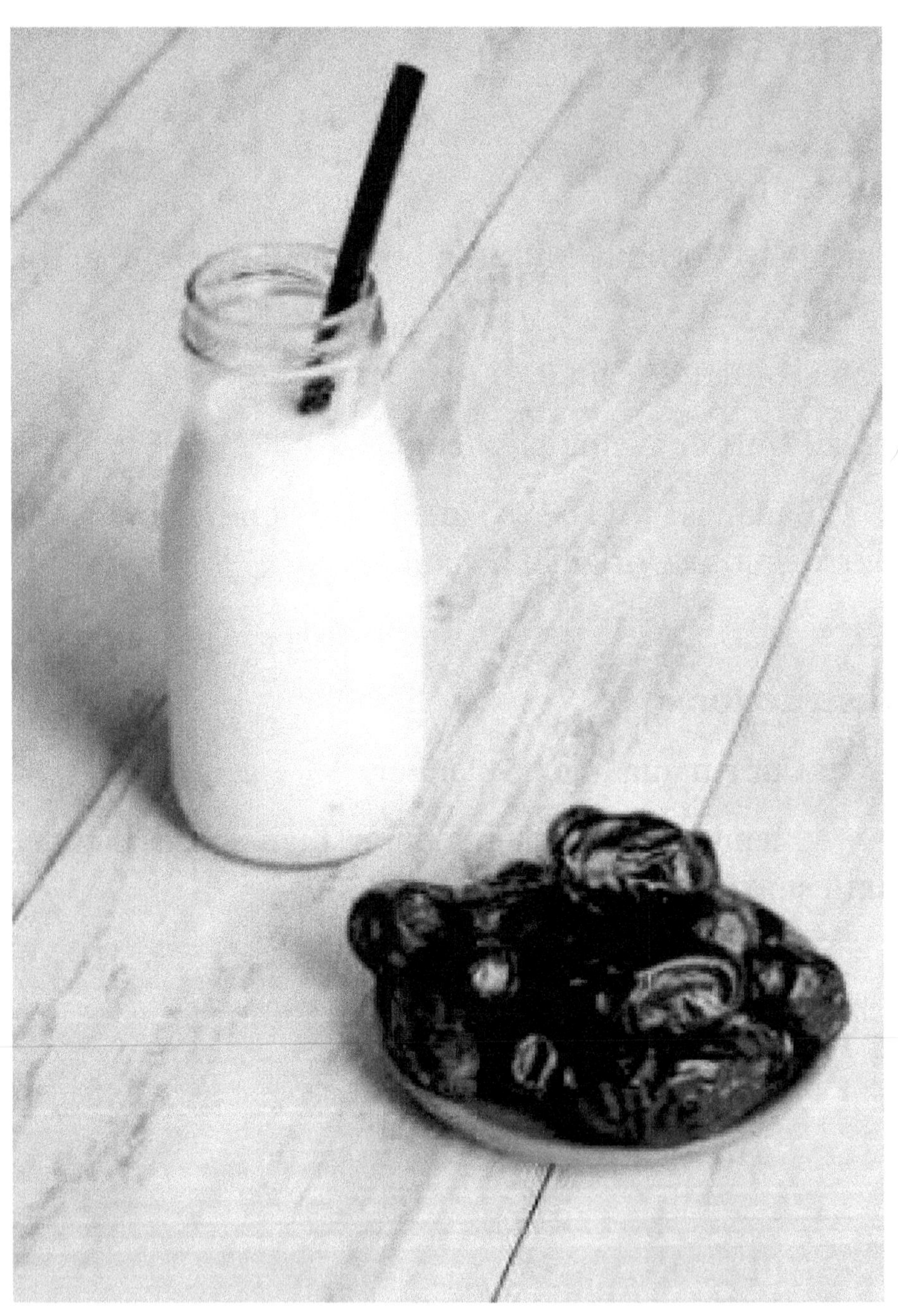

www.ingramcontent.com/pod-product-compliance
Lightning Source LLC
Chambersburg PA
CBHW061003050726
47592CB00003B/1329